PREFACE

The Tavistock Classics in the History of Psychiatry series meets a considerable need amongst academics, practitioners, and all those who are more broadly interested in the development of psychiatry. Psychiatry as a discipline has always paid considerable heed to its own founders, its history, and emergent traditions. It is one field in which the relevance of the past to the present does not diminish. There is a high professional awareness of the history of the subject, and many aspects of this are now benefiting from fruitful dialogue with the now rapidly expanding investigations of historians and historical sociologists.

Yet two factors greatly hamper our grasp of psychiatry's past. On the one hand, a considerable number of the formative texts in the rise of psychiatry are exceedingly difficult to obtain, even from libraries. As a small discipline in earlier centuries, many of the major works were published only in short runs, and many, even of the classics, have never been reprinted at all. This present series aims to overcome this problem, by making available a selection of such key works. Mostly they are books originally published in the English language; in other cases where the original language was, say, French or German, we are reprinting contemporary English translations; in a few cases, we hope to present entirely new translations of classic Continental works.

On the other hand, in many instances little is commonly known of the life and ideas of the authors of these texts, and their works have never been subjected to thorough analyses. Our intention in this series is to follow the model of the now defunct Dawson series of psychiatric reprints, edited and introduced by Richard Hunter and Ida Macalpine, now, alas, both dead, and to provide substantial scholarly introductions to each volume, based upon original research. Thus the book and its author will illuminate each other, and one will avoid the dilemma of a text isolated in an intellectual vacuum, or simply the accumulation of miscellaneous biographical data. It is our hope that this series will break new ground in the history of psychiatry, and secure a new readership for a number of illustrative works in psychiatry's rich and fascinating past.

OBSERVATIONS

ON

MANIACAL DISORDERS

Tavistock Classics
in the History of Psychiatry

GENERAL EDITORS:

W.F. Bynum and Roy Porter

Current interest in the history of psychiatry is growing rapidly both among
the psychiatric profession and social historians. This new series is designed to bring
back into print many classic documents from earlier centuries. Each reprint has
been chosen for the series because of its social and intellectual significance, and
includes a substantial introduction written by an eminent scholar in the history of
psychiatry.

Lifes Preservative Against Self-Killing (1637)
by John Sym (*ed.* Michael MacDonald)

Illustrations of Madness (1810)
by John Haslam (*ed.* Roy Porter)

An Essay . . . on Drunkenness (1804)
by Thomas Trotter (*ed.* Roy Porter)

OBSERVATIONS

ON

MANIACAL DISORDERS

BY

WILLIAM PARGETER

Edited with an Introduction by

Stanley W. Jackson

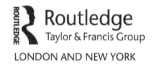

LONDON AND NEW YORK

First published 1988
by Routledge

2 Park Square, Milton Park, Abingdon, Oxfordshire OX14 4RN
711 Third Avenue, New York, NY 10017

First issued in paperback 2014

Routledge is an imprint of the Taylor and Francis Group, an informa business

British Library Cataloguing in Publication Data

Pargeter, William
  Observations on maniacal disorders.
  1. England. Man. Mental illness, history
  I. Title   II. Jackson, Stanley W.
  (Stanley Webber), *1920–*   II. Series
  616.89′00942

Library of Congress Cataloging in Publication Data

Pargeter, William, 1760–1810.
  Observations on maniacal disorders/Reverend William Pargeter:
edited with an introduction by Stanley W. Jackson.
    p.   cm. — (Tavistock classics in the history of psychiatry)
  Reprint. Originally published: Reading: W. Pargeter, 1792.
  Includes index.
  ISBN 978-0-415-00638-5 (hbk)
  ISBN 978-0-415-86748-1 (pbk)

    1. Manic-depressive psychoses—Early works to 1800.   I.
Jackson.
  Stanley W., 1920–   . II. Title   III. Series.
  [DNLM: WZ 290 P229o 1792F]
  RC516.P35 1988
  616.89′5—dc19
  DNLM/DLC   88–18630
  for Library of Congress   CIP

CONTENTS

v

INTRODUCTION

Stanley W. Jackson

Twentieth-century writings on the history of psychiatry have frequently suggested that a remarkable new approach to the care of insane persons emerged suddenly in the 1790s, coming almost out of the blue and associated with the names of Pinel and Tuke. Without taking anything away from the contributions of Pinel and Tuke, it is important to note that a new emphasis on the management of the mad, as distinct from 'physicking' them, was already under way. As will be seen in the final section of this Introduction, statements regarding this changing philosophy of the therapeutics of insanity had begun to appear during the eighteenth century, and there were numerous hints that some practitioners cared for their mad patients in ways constructively different than the received stereotypes of eighteenth-century care.[1]

In his *Observations on Maniacal Disorders*, William Pargeter (1760–1810), reflected this change in therapeutic philosophy.[2] In contrast to others who had written in this vein, he was not a madhouse proprietor advertising his services. He wrote without a vested interest in 'the trade in lunacy'.[3] He argued for humane care and efforts to gain the patient's confidence, and against 'chains and cords', 'beating', forcing remedies on patients, and the use of 'stupefying liquor' to 'drown their faculties'. As others had begun to do, he presented a series of case reports, but, different from his predecessors, he took some pains to detail just what he did to gain his patient's confidence and to promote in practical fashion what was increasingly being espoused as a therapeutic philosophy.

Just why Pargeter wrote this particular book, and wrote it when he did, is difficult to say with any certainty, but his Preface places him among those who were concerned to argue that George III's recent illness was a *symptomatic* or *febrile delirium* rather than a *maniacal disorder* (and thus a delirium without fever) as so many had thought. The nation had been set astir by the King's loss of reason in 1788, and the evolving eighteenth-century concerns regarding humane care for the mad received further support as a result of the 'royal malady'.[4] Pargeter was already interested in such matters, and had treated a number of mentally disturbed persons. But the English scene following the King's illness and recovery may well have provided the impetus that moved him to authorship, and to a work on 'maniacal disorders' in particular.[5] Pargeter's book supported his argument that the King had not been insane, and it implicitly argued against the severity of the care that he had received.

Pargeter's case for more benevolent care built on emerging trends, on a therapeutic philosophy already in the process of being articulated. But he was the first to support his case with clear evidence from his own clinical experience, to detail his technique in writing, and to illustrate in these ways what could be accomplished through humane 'management'.

Although not mentioned with any great frequency by his contemporaries, Pargeter's *Observations* was noted to be 'a very useful work: it contains much information' in the *Critical Review* in 1792,[6] and a German translation was published in Leipzig in 1793.[7] David Daniel Davis cited it favourably in his translator's Introduction to the English translation of Pinel's *Traité ... sur ... la Manie* in 1806.[8] Johann Christian Heinroth was warm in his praise in 1818, using Pargeter to illustrate the excellence of the English as practitioners in the treatment of 'disturbances of the soul'.[9] Emphasizing the practical value of Pargeter's *Observations*, Johannes Baptista Friedreich discussed his work at some length in 1830 in his history of the pathology and treatment of mental diseases.[10] Ernst von Feuchtersleben mentioned him briefly in 1845, and Daniel Hack Tuke took note of his work in 1882 and again in 1892.[11]

William Pargeter (1760–1810): biographical outline

William Pargeter[12] was an English physician of the late eighteenth century. As was the case with many eighteenth-century physicians, he came from a family of country clergymen. He was born in 1760, the son of Robert Pargeter (1726–90), BA (Oxon.), the rector of Stapleford in Hertfordshire, and the grandson of Robert Pargeter (1695–1741), MA (Oxon.), the vicar of Bloxham in Oxfordshire. He had an older brother, Robert (1759–1803), MA (Oxon.), about whom nothing is known except that he died in Kentish Town, and a younger brother, Philip (?1762–1839), who also studied medicine, practising first as a surgeon and apothecary at Wokingham near Reading, and later at Fordingbridge in Hampshire; and he had at least two sisters, about whom little is known. Nothing is known of Pargeter's early life until he entered Oxford University in January 1777, where he graduated as a BA from New College in February 1781.

At New College he was influenced by Martin Wall (1747–1824), Fellow of the College, physician to the Radcliffe Infirmary, and, from 1786 to his death, Lichfield Professor of Clinical Medicine at Oxford. Pargeter came to be a student of medicine there, and was one of the six founder-members of the Medical Society of Oxford, a student society in which he played a prominent role.[13] Wall is said to have introduced Pargeter to medicine and to have been responsible for his move, approximately two years after taking his degree at Oxford, to London and St Bartholomew's Hospital, where Wall had studied and where Pargeter remained a student until 1786. A fellow student at St Bartholomew's was John Haslam (1764–1844), who became the resident apothecary at Bethlehem Hospital (Bedlam) and an authority on mental disorders; and another contemporary there was Andrew Marshal (1742–1813), who was to argue so strongly that madness was always connected with disease of the brain and its membranes. For none of the three is there any extant record of the time spent at St Bartholomew's.[14]

In November 1786 he graduated as MD from Marischal College, Aberdeen, by the customary method of producing letters of recommendation and paying a fee of 25 pounds. His letters of support came from Drs Martin Wall and William Austin (1754–93), the latter having been Professor of Chemistry and Physician at the Radcliffe Infirmary during Pargeter's time at Oxford, a fellow member of the Medical Society of Oxford, and, in 1786, having been elected Physician to St Bartholomew's Hospital.

Pargeter then practised in London until at least 1787. What little evidence there is from then until 1795 suggests that he was not far from Oxford and associates him with Reading. His *Observations* was published at Reading in 1792, and that same year *The Reading Mercury* in its advertisement of his book referred to him as being 'of Reading'. His brother, Philip, was in practice near there, and it seems likely that he too practised in that region. In his preface to *Observations*, he thanked 'Lord *Lichfield*'s Clinical Professor' (Dr Martin Wall) for the use of his library in the preparation of the book, thus placing himself in the vicinity of Oxford.

In 1795 Pargeter's only other medical work was published in London. *Formulae Medicamentorum Selectae* was a 58-page book in duodecimo, published anonymously, but the author's identity readily betrayed by the title page's 'By the author of *Maniacal Observations*' and further suggested by the advertisement for *Observations* at the end of the work. Known by a single copy in the Library of the Pharmaceutical Society, it has been described as 'of interest only as a forerunner of pocket hospital pharmacopoeias'.[15] Reviewers were not kind, faulting its Latin and minimizing its value. Pargeter brought his medical career to a close that same year, taking Holy Orders and, as the Reverend William Pargeter, entering the Royal Navy as a chaplain,[16] in which capacity he served until 1802.

After two other brief assignments, on 12 December 1795 he was posted, as her chaplain, to HMS *Alexander*, on which he served until September 1800, except for a brief period that last summer. In August 1796 Captain (later Sir) Alexander John Ball took command of the ship, and at the beginning of May 1798 she was sent into the Mediterranean under the orders of Horatio Nelson in HMS *Vanguard*. The destruction of the French fleet which followed on 1 August 1798, at the Battle of the Nile, was the only major engagement Pargeter saw; of the *Alexander*'s crew of 590, 14 were killed and 58 wounded. After that battle the ship blockaded Malta for two years. When Malta capitulated on 4 September 1800, and Captain Ball went ashore in command of the militia (later he became Governor of Malta), Pargeter followed him as chaplain to the island's garrison. Later that year General Abercromby visited Malta as commander-in-chief in the Mediterranean. Then, on 28 March 1801, he was killed at the Battle of Alexandria, and his body was brought back to Malta for burial. Pargeter's memorial sermon on this occasion was his third and last published work.[17]

Introduction by Stanley W. Jackson

After a time the climate in Malta began 'not agreeing with his constitution' (*Gentleman's Magazine*, 1810), so when Alexander called on December 26, 1801, he took the opportunity to rejoin his old ship; and when her company was disbanded at Portsmouth on August 26, 1802, he retired from the Navy on pension.[18]

Pargeter then returned to his home county of Oxfordshire, staying first in the city of Oxford and later moving to the village of Bloxham which had been his grandfather's parish. There he lived out his remaining years, apparently not resuming the practice of medicine, and dying on 17 May 1810.

Mania: the term and the disorder

In classical Greece mania often seems to have meant madness in a relatively loose and general sense, but at times it had the more specific meaning of raving madness. Gradually mania came to be viewed as one of the three traditional forms of madness in ancient medicine, the others being melancholia and phrenitis. These three disorders were categorized under diseases of the head, with mania and melancholia characterized as chronic diseases without fever and contrasted with phrenitis as an acute disease with fever. Usually mania meant a state of derangement associated with severe excitement and often wild behaviour. But, while many used the term in this narrower sense, frequently enough to confuse a modern reader it was also used as a generic term for madness or insanity. In these latter instances, a discussion of mania would often include both cases of raving madness and cases of dejected or melancholic madness, sometimes clearly differentiated as separate disorders and sometimes with a considerable blurring of any boundaries between them; and sometimes the term mania was used to refer to an even wider variety of disorders that today would be considered psychotic in nature. Thus the mania of the Ancients may at times be readily reconciled with our modern use of the term, and at other times not very well at all.

In the medicine of ancient Greece and Rome, and for many centuries thereafter, mania as raving madness and melancholia as dejected madness were intimately associated with one another, sometimes as clearly contrasted chronic disorders without fever, sometimes as contrasted conditions within a chapter on mania or a chapter on melancholia, and sometimes not at all well differentiated from one another. There were those who argued that they were essentially one disease, and there were those who argued that this was not the case. And there were those who maintained that melancholia might worsen and become mania, or that mania might lessen in severity and become merely melancholia. Although these various connections between mania and melancholia surely have their place in the historical background of the nineteenth-century's circular insanity and the twentieth-century's manic-depressive disease and bipolar disorder, one must be cautious about reading modern meanings into such connections.[19]

In the second century AD, in what are probably the earliest extant accounts of mania that provide any significant detail, first Soranus of Ephesus (early second century), and then Aretaeus of Cappadocia (*c.* AD 150), left descriptions that are clearly akin to modern mania, and discussions that reflect the tendency to connect mania with melancholia. For Soranus,[20] mania involved an impairment of reason with delusions; fluctuating states of anger and merriment, although sometimes of sadness and futility and sometimes 'an overpowering fear of things which are quite harmless'; 'continual wakefulness, the veins are distended, cheeks flushed, and body hard and abnormally strong'; and a tendency for there to be 'attacks alternating with periods of remission'. In his chapter on mania, Aretaeus[21] observed that it was 'a chronic derangement of mind, without fever'; provided lively descriptions of excited clinical states, some of them joyous and grandiose, and some of them angry and dangerous; noted that delusions were common; and mentioned insomnia. Although each took some pains to differentiate mania from various other forms of madness, for both Soranus and Aretaeus it is clear that mania included a wider range of conditions than the twentieth century would group under this term, and yet it clearly included conditions similar to our mania. It was predominantly a matter of excited states, delusions, wild behaviour, grandiosity, and related affects. Another point worth noting is that each of these authors placed his chapter on mania immediately next to his chapter on melancholia in his book on chronic diseases. This arrangement as adjacent chapters, either in works on chronic diseases or in sections on diseases of the head, was to become a long-standing tradition; and the commonest exception was when they were treated in a single chapter, with the two accounts interwoven to varying extents and the title sometimes mania, sometimes melancholia, and sometimes as a combination.

Also found in Aretaeus' comments on mania are the seeds of an explanation that was to be associated with mania for many centuries to come. He stated that mania was 'something hot and dry in cause'.[22] Later in the second century AD, Galen (131–201) referred to mania as a pathological excitement caused by a biting and hot humour, the yellow bile.[23] In the humoral theory taken up by Galen from his predecessors and subscribed to by his successors over the next 1500 years, mania was thought to be caused by yellow bile, the hot and dry humour; and, in the associated theory of qualities systematized by Galen, mania came to be conceived of as a hot and dry disease and as the result of hot and dry causes. A related humoral explanation was based on the notion that the various humours might become overheated and burnt, the result being a hot and dry humour termed adust or burnt black bile. Contrasted with the natural black bile, a cold and dry humour thought to cause melancholia, this unnatural black bile was put forward by some authorities as the cause of excited or raving forms of madness, sometimes called mania and sometimes an excited type of melancholia.[24]

Throughout the medieval era and into the seventeenth century, these patterns of clinical description and explanation continued much the same. Mania continued to imply primarily excited or raving states of madness, and melancholia dejected states of madness. Although most authors during these centuries conceived of them as two separate diseases, the occasional author cited Aretaeus or Alexander of Tralles (AD 525–605) as a basis for asserting a more intimate connection between them; but the connection suggested was usually that of melancholia as the earlier stage and milder form of madness, and mania as the later stage and more serious or advanced form.

In the latter half of the seventeenth century, Thomas Willis (1621–75) followed the common practice of presenting mania and melancholia as two distinct diseases, but he employed a metaphor that could be taken to imply two aspects of a single process. With the English translation using the term *raving* as the generic term, much as many predecessors had used *madness*, he defined melancholia as 'a raving without a Feavour or fury, joined with fear and sadness'.[25] Mania, too, was 'without a Feavour', but it entailed

> a Fury ... and Boldness, Strength, and that they are still unwearied with any labours, and suffer pains unhurt .... *Madmen* are not as *Melancholicks*, sad and fearful, but audacious and very confident, so that they shun almost no dangers, and attempt all the most difficult things that are.[26]

Here Willis was mentioning elements noted in many a previous clinical description of mania. Then, at the beginning of his chapter on mania, he stated that these two disorders were so much akin that they

> often change, and pass from one into the other; for the *Melancholick* disposition growing worse, brings on *Fury*; and *Fury* or *Madness* growing less hot, oftentimes ends in a *Melancholick* disposition. These two, like smoke and flame, mutually receive and give place one to another. And indeed, if in *Melancholy* the Brain and Animal Spirits are said to be darkened with fume, and a thick obscurity; In *Madness*, they seem to be all as it were of an open burning of flame.[27]

With Willis it is important to note that chemical explanations became prominent in attempting to account for mental disorders, including mania. Reflecting trends dating back to Paracelsus in the previous century and furthered by Van Helmont and others in the seventeenth century, he challenged the four classical humours, and replaced them with the five 'Principles of Chymists' (spirit, sulphur, salt, water, earth) in his explanations of disease. In a complex scheme of pathogenesis, he used these chemical principles to account for disturbances in the animal spirits, his effective agent in nervous transmission, for which the nervous liquor served as the vehicle as it, in turn, made its way along the subtly porous nerves. In his view, in mania the animal spirits shifted from their normal '*Saline*' nature to a '*Sulphureous-Saline* disposition, like to *Stygian*-Water', and so, like the 'Particles of *Stygian*-Water', they became 'highly active and unquiet'.[28]

Introduction by Stanley W. Jackson

Also of significance to the history of mania was Willis's differentiation of melancholia into two types: a *universal* type in which 'the distemper'd are *Delirious* as to all things, or at least as to most; so that they judge truly almost of no subject'; and a *particular* type in which 'they imagine amiss in one or two particular cases, but for the most part in other things, they have their notions not very incongruous'.[29] During the eighteenth century this concept came to be used somewhat differently, with *universal insanity* referring to mania and *particular* or *partial insanity* to melancholia.

Hermann Boerhaave (1668–1738) began his section on mania by saying that

> if Melancholy increases so far, that from the great Motion of the Liquid of the Brain, the Patient be thrown into a wild Fury, it is call'd *Madness*. Which differs only in Degree from the sorrowful kind of Melancholy, is its Offspring, produced from the same Causes, and cured almost by the same Remedies.

To these comments he added a familiar list of symptoms: 'the Patient generally shews a great Strength of the Muscles, an incredible Wakefulness, a bearing to a wonder of Cold and Hunger, frightful Fancies, Endeavors to bite Men like Wolves, or Dogs, etc'.[30] It should be noted that the term *madness* here meant mania, a common enough practice in English, but also that it reflected the English translator's choice of terms for Boerhaave's *mania* in Latin, a very common practice. By Boerhaave's time a trend was under way that would separate hypochondriasis out from melancholia in the view of many, with the former as a less severe, often non-mad, disorder.[31] Boerhaave's version of this trend was to conceive of them as though they were two degrees of severity within a single illness, and then he discussed mania as the next degree of severity beyond melancholia. Thus, while he presented mania as a separate disorder, he thought in terms of hypochondriasis-melancholia-mania as a continuum of increasing severity.

To appreciate Boerhaave's ideas on pathogenesis, it is important to note that, along with Archibald Pitcairn (1652–1713) and Friedrich Hoffmann (1660–1742), he was in the vanguard of those who introduced mechanical explanations into his considerations of mental disorder.[32] The humoral theory was being abandoned, but the newer iatrochemical notions did not replace it for very long.

xvii

Introduction by Stanley W. Jackson

On mania, Boerhaave stated that it was 'produced from the same Causes' as melancholia.[33] He thought that the various precipitating factors that might occasion melancholia did so through the elimination or reduction of the 'most moveable' parts of the blood and a slowing of the movement of the rest of the blood, and that this led to the development of a sort of atrabiliary sludge that led to the melancholic symptoms.[34] Boerhaave was much less clear regarding the pathogenesis of mania. He seemed to imply that this slowing of the blood and development of an atrabiliary sludge went even further in mania, and yet he also attributed mania to a 'great Motion of the Liquid of the Brain'.[35] As he mentioned both instances of mania that followed in the wake of an exhausting illness and other instances 'in strong, hale, youthful, plethoric People of a hot Constitution', perhaps these two contrasting types were thought to be accounted for by these two contrasting schemes of pathogenesis.[36]

In much the same vein as Boerhaave, and often directly influenced by him, a good many eighteenth-century authors discussed mania and melancholia as intimately connected: as two disorders that might shift from one into the other, or as related to one another on a continuum of severity, or even as 'one species of Disorder'. And it was common to cite 'an excessive Congestion of the Blood in the Brain' as the essential cause.[37] By the latter half of the century it had also become usual to conceive of melancholia as partial insanity, i.e., the derangement limited to a single idea or a small number of related ideas, and of mania as universal insanity, i.e., the derangement extended through much of the person's thinking. Thus a continuum of increasingly disordered intellectual functioning became another version of the idea of melancholia degenerating into mania or worsening to become mania.

The views of William Cullen (1710–90) on mania bring us close to the end of the eighteenth century and up to the eve of Pargeter's own work. He was one of the most influential medical men in the latter half of the century, and he was the particular authority whom Pargeter cited as the main source of his nosological considerations and his theories for explaining mania. As did other well-known nosologists of that era, such as De Sauvages and Linnaeus, Cullen clearly distinguished mania as universal insanity from melancholia as partial insanity in his *Nosology*.[38] He did the same in his *First Lines of the Practice of Physic*, although there he was doubtful as to whether the insanity was always only partial in melancholia.[39]

In his chapter on melancholia in the *First Lines*, Cullen referred to mania as 'often no other than a higher degree of melancholia'.[40] Then, in his chapter on mania, he mentioned 'those causes of mania which arise in consequence of a melancholia which had previously long subsisted'.[41] This latter category, though, was no more than a sub-set of cases within what he termed *Mental Mania (Mania mentalis)* which resulted 'altogether from passion of the mind'. He also recognized two other species of mania, *Corporeal Mania (Mania corporea)* and *Obscure Mania (Mania obscura)*, the former resulting 'from an evident fault of the body' and the latter having been 'not preceded by any passion of the mind or evident fault of the body'.[42] The more frequent causes stemmed from 'violent emotions or passions of the mind', and so belonged to the species *Mental Mania*.[43] As to his clinical description, in contrast to melancholia which he had suggested was often associated with false judgement on a single subject, he stated that in mania

> more commonly the mind rambles from one subject to another with an equally false judgment concerning the most part of them; and as at the same time there is commonly a false associa- tion, this increases the confusion of ideas, and therefore the false judgments. What for the most part more especially distinguishes the disease is a hurry of mind, in pursuing any thing like a train of thought, and in running from one train of thought to another. Maniacal persons are in general very irasc- ible; but what more particularly produces their angry emotions, is, that their false judgments lead to some action which is always pushed with impetuosity and violence; when this is interrupted or restrained, they break out into violent anger and furious violence against every person near them, and upon every thing that stands in the way of their impetuous will.[44]

He also noted that it was common for there to be

> an unusual force in all the voluntary motions; and an insensi- bility or resistance of the force of all impressions, and parti- cularly a resistance of the powers of sleep, of cold, and even of hunger; though indeed in many instances a voracious appetite takes place.[45]

Introduction by Stanley W. Jackson

To grasp Cullen's ideas on the pathogenesis of mania, one must first consider the basic theories that informed his physiology and pathophysiology. He shifted from the heart and the vascular system that were central to the physiology of most of his eighteenth-century predecessors, to the brain and the nervous system as the basic elements in his own physiology; and with this shift he abandoned the hydraulics and the hydrodynamic principles of the Boerhaavian system, both for the immediate functions of the nervous system and for its new functions as a source of primary causes for physiological activities in general. Central to Cullen's neural explanations was a system of forces and a nerve fluid reflecting elements of both Haller's physiology and Newton's speculative mechanics for the nervous system.[46] He rejected any notions of the brain as a secretory organ and of hollow nerves with a circulatory nerve fluid. He cautiously put forward the idea of 'nervous power', but ultimately chose to refer to it as a nerve fluid. This fluid was inherent in the nerves and mediated the transmission of oscillatory or vibratory motions; and he conceived of it as one of a group of imperceptible and imponderable fluids that were modifications of Newton's aether.[47] On these foundations Cullen constructed a theory of disease in which the ideas of 'excitement' and 'collapse' were used extensively in the discussion of both normal and abnormal states. Excitement referred to conditions ranging from the normal state of being awake, to a pathological extreme such as mania, and collapse referred to conditions ranging from the normal state of sleeping, to pathological extremes such as syncope and death. He conceived of excitement and collapse as states of increased and decreased mobility of the nervous power or nervous fluid in the brain whose effects were felt throughout the nervous system.[48] Against this background, Cullen thought of normal mental function as entailing a relatively even distribution of controlled amounts of excitement through the various parts of the brain. In the case of delirium, by which he meant disordered judgement, he postulated inequalities in the degree of excitement in different parts of the brain. The forms of delirium without fever were the insanities, namely, mania and melancholia.[49] Mania involved

> a considerable and unusual excess in the excitement of
> the brain, especially with respect to the animal [i.e. mental]

functions; and it appears at the same time to be manifestly in some measure unequal, as it very often takes place with respect to these functions alone.

That is, Cullen subscribed to a 'doctrine of increased and unequal excitement' as the pathophysiological essence of mania.[50]

Pargeter's book

As Pargeter made quite clear in his Preface and in the early pages of his book, his basic physiological theory and his notions of pathophysiology were taken directly from 'the *Professor*' – Dr William Cullen of Edinburgh.[51] He adopted Cullen's ideas of *excitement* and *collapse*, each referring to a particular direction of morbid change in 'the tone of the brain' and 'the motion of the nervous fluid'. Using the term 'delirium', as Cullen had, to mean disordered judgement or functioning of the intellect, he cited 'the delirium occurring at falling asleep, or at first waking out of sleep' as instances of Cullen's thesis that delirium was the result of 'an *unequal excitement* of the different parts' of the brain, with the implication that these two instances were temporary and within normal limits. This was in contrast to 'the perfect exercise of our intellectual faculties' which required 'some *equality* in the *excitement* of every part of the brain'. More severe and less temporary instances of delirium entailed 'an *uncommonly encreased excitement* of the brain ... a principal circumstance in *Mania*', which view Pargeter thought was 'confirmed by the increased impetus of the blood, a common cause of too great *excitement* of the brain inducing *delirium* in phrenitis, and fever'. In contrast to phrenitis as an acute delirium with fever, mania was a chronic delirium without fever. He also noted that normal functioning

> depends upon a certain degree or measure in the force and velocity with which ... *ideas* take place, and therefore it is, that every cause of hurry throws us into confusion, which is a momentary and slight degree of *Mania*.

He noted that 'every sudden emotion is liable to have this effect, and some emotions produce it more permanently'.[52]

Against this background Pargeter portrayed the clinical picture of mania. He observed that 'in most instances of *Mania*, in every instance of the *Mania furibunda*, a violently *encreased excitement* is manifest from the increase of strength and vigour which takes place'. He then proceeded to relate other symptoms of mania to increased excitement. The severe insomnia, the resistance to the effects of both natural and medical sedative agents, and the insensibility to the effects of cold, were each related to a resistance 'to impressions of every kind'. He referred to 'the *fury* of Maniacs' as a further 'mark of a strongly *excited state* of the mind, and therefore of the brain', and related this to the more short-lived states of excitement associated with 'paroxysms of anger, which is *furor brevis*'.[53] Later in the book, he elaborated, noting that such patients

> become restless – more loquacious – haughty and supercilious in their demeanour – are suspicious – fickle – captious and inquisitive about trifles – have a furious aspect – redness of the eyes – a quick sense of hearing – are irritable, particularly at meals – they entertain an inveterate aversion to particular persons.

As the disorder worsened, they would 'hallow – swear – pray – sing – cry – laugh, and talk lasciviously, almost in the same instant'.[54] Thus mania was essentially an excited form of insanity or a raving madness for Pargeter, as for most of his predecessors and contemporaries.

In a manner also quite typical for his time, Pargeter viewed melancholia as closely connected to mania, and he wrote of these two conditions varyingly, sometimes as though they were distinct disorders, and sometimes as though both were subsumed under the rubric 'maniacal disorders' or mania. At times his language in discussing the two conditions could be confusing to the modern reader. Like mania, melancholia was a form of madness, a delirium without fever. Following Cullen once again, he referred to mania as *Insania Universalis*, with the implication that melancholia was *Insania Particularis*. The former term meant that the person was delirious or delusional on many or most matters, and the latter meant that the person was delusional on one or two subjects while being quite rational on other matters.[55] Although a continuum of severity may or may not have been implied here, such a relationship had commonly been an explicit one since Boerhaave, with mania differing from melancholia only in degree for many authorities; and many an earlier author had observed that melancholia might worsen and turn into mania, while conceiving of them as distinct disorders. Pargeter clearly thought of melancholia as a milder form of madness that might well worsen and develop into mania. Early in his book he stated that 'the doctrine of *Mania* includes in some degree that of *Melancholia*, consequently they cannot be *generically* different'.[56] Then, at intervals throughout the book, he used the terms *Mania tranquilla* and *Mania innocua* as synonyms for *Melancholia*, and he contrasted these terms to *Mania furibunda* meaning the traditional *Mania* or raving madness. His clinical picture for melancholia included thoughtfulness, profound taciturnity, a fondness for solitude, obstinacy, loss of appetite, insomnia, constipation, low-spiritedness, and lamenting, weeping, and sighing heavily, without any apparent cause.[57] His commonest practice was to use *Mania tranquilla* (or *Melancholia*) and to indicate that it was quite different from *Mania furibunda* (or *Mania*), but that there was always the danger that the former might worsen and develop into the latter. Interestingly, in detailing the treatment of one patient, he stated that 'by *management*, *Mania furibunda* was evidently and happily reduced to *Mania tranquilla*'.[58]

In considering the causes of mania, Pargeter briefly mentioned 'the proximate causes' that occasioned the disturbed states of excitement in the brain that he associated with mania. 'The principal of these' were '*various topical affections of the brain – watry effusions – obscure shirri – preternatural ossifications – and numerous causes of increased impetus of the blood in the head*'.[59] He then postulated that 'the *primary* cause of Insanity' was 'a certain morbid or *irritating* principle or quality' of the nervous fluid ('or electrical aura, as some style it') in 'the nervous tubuli'.[60] This idea was almost certainly another reflection of Cullen's thinking, although Pargeter's statement that the nervous fluid was 'secreted by the cerebrum and cerebellum', for all its currency at that time, was apparently not a notion subscribed to by Cullen. Proceeding to 'the ordinary *remote* causes', under 'those acting on the mind' he discussed 'sudden and violent emotions, or passions', such as fear, anger, and joy, and 'all the strong and durable depressing passions – *Grief, sadness, despair*'; and, still under '*remote* causes ... acting on the mind', he noted that '*intense study* and *application of mind*, is one of the most common causes' and also cited '*meditation*'.[61] Further on 'the ordinary *remote* causes', he reviewed 'those whose first operation is on the body' – '*poisons*', such as '*opium*' and '*mercurial medicines*'; '*suppressed evacuations* and *repelled eruptions*', probably by 'causing a determination of blood to the brain'; and 'an high degree of *lust* and *salacity*'.[62] Finally, he commented that 'to these *remote* causes ... others may be assigned as *auxiliaries* in spreading the unhappy disease'. Here he mentioned 'the *Luxury* of the times'; '*Fanaticism*', meaning 'religious *enthusiasm*', specially indicating 'the *doctrines* of the *Methodists*'; and 'a *Lunatic Ancestry*'.[63]

On the 'ordinary *remote* causes', Pargeter was taking note of possible causes that were familiar ones in eighteenth-century writings. Regarding '*Luxury*', he was sounding a familiar note, indicating the pernicious effects of an overly indulgent or otherwise decadent way of life. This theme was commonly mentioned by eighteenth-century medical authors when discussing both mental and physical disorders. In light of the emergence of the concept of *degeneration* in nineteenth-century views on the etiology of mental disorders, it is of interest that he alleged that there had been a downward or deteriorating drift over the generations and referred to it as 'this degeneracy'.[64] 'Religious *enthusiasm*' had been taken note of in association with melancholia during the seventeenth and eighteenth centuries, sometimes as a type of melancholia and sometimes as a cause of melancholia. In the eighteenth century, though, there was a shift toward more allegations that such *enthusiasm* was associated with mania and fewer with melancholia.[65] As to 'a *Lunatic Ancestry*', a hereditary predisposition was a familiar enough notion that it was mentioned by William Buchan (1729–1805) in his *Domestic Medicine*, but heredity was to be emphasized much more in nineteenth-century considerations of causes.[66]

Pargeter's discussion of the causes of mania certainly included some factors that were *not* physical agents and would today be considered pyschological in nature. Further, he stated that

> many cases of *Mania* are short and transitory, and admit of very sudden changes – these certainly are not dependant on any *organic* affection – others continue through life; it is equally improbable, that any *organic* affection is here present.

Although he concluded that no organ disease could be identified, he thought that the tendency to recurrence suggested 'a peculiar affection of the brain' of an uncertain nature. This view was akin to the notion of a functional disorder a century later, in which undemonstrated physiological dysfunction was suspected even though no somatic pathology could be found. He then went on to maintain that

> there must indeed be in every case of *Mania*, in all probability, some peculiar corporeal morbid state, with which that peculiar state of mind is connected; and it is more than probable, that the corporeal part affected is the brain.[67]

Essentially, we have here the credo enunciated by Wilhelm Griesinger (1817–68) fifty years later.[68] After surveying various authorities on the post-mortem examination of the brain in cases of mania, Pargeter commented that 'most of the *anatomists* seem to consider the *preternatural hardness* of the cerebrum and cerebellum, as the only circumstance that deserved particular notice in the brains of the *Maniacal* patients they had dissected'. But the experience of a few authorities, and his own limited post-mortem experience, left him with the 'opinion, that no true judgment can be formed from any morbid appearances which the brain may exhibit on dissection, because it will be impossible to determine whether those appearances are *causes* or *effects*'.[69]

When it came to the treatment of mania, Pargeter had much to say that was familiar and traditional. To reduce the excessive excitement, he mentioned, as *internal remedies*, abstinence from food, various evacuant remedies (bleeding, cathartics, emetics, discharges by setons, and sternutatories), blistering plasters, and 'medicines of the sedative class' (camphor, opium, musk, and hyoscyamus).[70] Again to counter the untoward excitement, he took note of various *external remedies*, such as cold for 'its sedative power' (a bonnet of snow or ice to the head, cold baths, ducking in cold water), various other applications to the head, and music for its soothing effects.[71] On music, Pargeter provided an interesting short essay on its usefulness, referring to it as 'the *Nepenthes* of the Gods'.[72] Each of these, and usually some combination thereof, had been frequently prescribed for maniacal disorders, and were common therapeutic measures in the eighteenth century. Parenthetically, he intermittently made briefer references to the therapeutic measures to be used when it was a case of *Mania tranquilla* or melancholia, reflecting the familiar contrast of energizing a dejected person rather than calming an excited one. Pargeter discussed these various remedies against a backdrop of significant conviction as to the importance of *management* in the care and cure of the mad. At times he apparently conceived of *management* as sufficient for the recovery of a mad person, but in other cases he viewed it as an approach by which the physician would be 'greatly assisted in the employment of other remedies'.[73] As we shall see in the following section ('Moral management and moral treatment'), though, he clearly valued *management* over physick.

What were the grounds on which Pargeter based his *Observations*, just outlined above? He carefully constructed this work on the basis of a significant familiarity with the relevant medical literature, but he also gave considerable attention to clinical cases as he proceeded. He noted in his Preface that, 'of the authors whose sentiments I have adopted, some I have mentioned, and others I could not call to my recollection'.[74] But, in addition to his carefully acknowledged indebtedness to Cullen, he actually cited many other medical authors, both ancient and contemporary, in appropriate and knowledgeable ways. Further, he also graced his text with many an apt literary quotation. As to the clinical material, he outlined eight cases of his own, half of which fitted the diagnosis of *Mania furibunda* (or mania) and half of which were more in the direction of *Mania tranquilla* (or melancholia), although he indicated that some of the latter group had been saved by treatment from worsening into *Mania furibunda*. He also cited one case where he had merely been called in as a consultant and another case that he had attended along with Dr Monro.[75] To illustrate specially dramatic delusions, he described a case from Wanley[76] and another from Lemnius.[77] In his discussion of cathartics, he cited the legendary account of the daughters of Proteus who were cured by Melampus;[78] he mentioned a case of van Helmont's to illustrate the value of plunging a patient into cold water;[79] he referred to the cure of Saul's melancholia in his discussion of the therapeutic value of music;[80] he outlined a case from Perfect as an example of *'arrogant Insanity'*;[81] he mentioned a case cited by Bonet where a cure had been affected by the transfusion of the blood of a calf;[82] he described two cases of Mead's to illustrate Mead's thesis that the onset of madness might cure an already existing disease;[83] and here and there he introduced clinical snippets from the writings of others to enrich the meaning of a point he was making.

Moral management and moral treatment

Pargeter's book contains some novel passages, particularly when one considers the alleged state of the care of mad persons around the time when it was published. If it had been published ten years later one might reasonably assume that he knew something about the emergence of *moral treatment* at the York Retreat, or that he had read Pinel's *Traité ... sur ... la Manie*, or, perhaps, that he had become aware of Chiarugi's work in Florence. But in 1792 the Retreat had not yet begun its work, Pinel had not yet taken up his post at the Bicêtre, and Chiarugi's work was unknown in Great Britain. Thus it might be thought that Pargeter had adumbrated some of the ideas that came to be associated with the names of William Tuke (1732–1822), Philippe Pinel (1745–1826), and Vincenzo Chiarugi (1759–1820).

Pargeter began his section on treatment as follows:

> The chief reliance in the cure of insanity must be rather on *management* than medicine. The *government* of maniacs is an art, not be be acquired without long experience, and frequent and attentive observation. Although it has been of late years much advanced, it is still capable of improvement.[84]

He then cited several cases 'to demonstrate what advantages may be accomplished by the art of *management*', and prefaced his consideration of other therapeutic measures with the statement, 'when a physician has gained this important point, (I mean the art of *management*) he will be greatly assisted in the employment of other remedies'.[85] Further, in the case descriptions offered to support these assertions, Pargeter indicated that he had had some practical experience with insane patients, and he provided some detail as to what he meant by 'management'.[86] In fact, these case reports were the first practical accounts, as distinct from the enunciation of general principles, of some of the psychological measures undertaken in the name of 'management'. Nevertheless, for all the fact that he wrote before the time of Tuke and Pinel, and for all that he was the first to detail the measures he took, he was not really original in his views.

In eighteenth-century literature on the care of the mad, there are clear indications that the above trend was already under way. Medications, bleeding, and various other forms of 'physicking' had long been traditional in the care of insane patients, and they continued to be mentioned regularly throughout the eighteenth century in addressing questions of how the mad should be treated. But, increasingly during that century, mention was made of the importance of attention to *management* as well as to physic in treating such patients. A particularly noteworthy example of this trend was that of William Battie (1703–76), who stated that

> the regimen in this [i.e., madness] is perhaps of more importance than in any distemper. It was the saying of a very eminent practitioner in such cases *that management did much more than medicine*; and repeated experience has convinced me that confinement alone is oftentimes sufficient, but always so necessary, that without it every method hitherto devised for the cure of Madness would be ineffectual.[87]

And, as we see, he made it clear that such a view was not new with him. Then, in a volume that was a response to 'the undeserved censures, which Dr Battie has thrown upon my predecessors', John Monro (1715–91), physician to Bethlehem Hospital, manifested very similar views. In the *Advertisement* to this work, he stated that 'the cure of that disorder [i.e., madness] depends on *management* as much as *medicine*',[88] and then wrote at some length on that subject under the heading, *Of the regimen and cure of madness*, indicating that Battie's 'very eminent practitioner in such cases' was probably Monro's late father and predecessor at Bethlehem Hospital, James Monro (1680–1752). On management, he commented as follows:

> As by *regimen* I presume is meant the *management* necessary for the cure of madness, I am thoroughly sensible, it is a point of the last importance, and in which the judgment and knowledge of the physician are of the utmost consequence.
> ... the *management* requisite for it [i.e., the treatment of madness] was never to be learned, but from observation ...

Management is universally allowed to be of the greatest moment, but other persons besides the physician must be concerned in this part, though they are to act under his direction; it may therefore be expected, that what we meet with on this head will be suited to common capacities, that it may be rendered more useful to the publick in general.[89]

Monro then referred to Battie's recommendations regarding confinement, healthful atmosphere, restriction from disturbing visitors, cleanliness, sound diet, and constructive management of the environment for insane patients, adding scathingly that these matters had occupied 'no farther than two pages, while the less important part of *medicine* takes up very near thirty'.[90] After considerable elaboration on Battie's themes as crucial elements of the care and management of the insane, Monro concluded with the following:

With regard to *management*, it is sometimes of consequence to know the *cause* of the disorder; not so much to direct us in the choice of medicines, as in the manner of conducting ourselves towards the patient: every one is not to be accosted in the same manner, some are to be commanded, others are to be soothed into compliance, but we should endeavour in every instance to gain their good opinion. It is impossible to be so full on this subject, as not to leave many things unsaid; much will depend upon the care and attention of the physician, whose method must vary according to the complaints of his patients; in this branch, neglect or ignorance will admit of no excuse: and I am very sure that *management* has not yet reached the perfection of which it is capable.[91]

Thus Pargeter's comments on *management* reflected a trend that already had a significant eighteenth-century history, which history he was almost certainly aware of[92] and to which he added his own opinion and his own clinical experience in his *Observations*. The York Retreat, Pinel, and Chiarugi, each came to play an important part in the advancing of that trend, each adding a body of experience and opinion that furthered the humane elements in it, even when one discounts for the later mythologizing of their contributions. Pargeter's contribution helps to make clearer the evolving context in which their work emerged and some aspects of its heritage.

Introduction by Stanley W. Jackson

What did *management* mean in these various eighteenth-century contexts? For one thing, the term itself referred to managing, training, or directing, as in the case of persons or animals. But, in medical writings, it had come to be used as a synonym for *regimen*, which had for many centuries meant the proper attention to the six non-naturals (air, exercise and rest, sleep and wakefulness, food and drink, excretion and retention of superfluities, and the passions or perturbations of the soul) in the interest of maintaining health in well persons or returning sick persons to health. In the case of the sick, this proper attention to the regimen by the physician (and others) entailed the retraining of the sick person in the direction of health. Guided by the principle of contraries, the goal was to return the person from sickness's imbalance in one or more of these factors to a healthful balance. As the term *management* came into use during the eighteenth century, it included just such traditional attention to the environment, to diet, to physical activity, and to the modification of untoward perturbations of the soul; and it gradually came to mean those aspects of medical care other than medications, blood-letting, and the like. The attention to the passions or perturbations of the soul had long entailed efforts to influence affective extremes back toward a happy medium, but these were now joined by the use of emotional states opposite to the disturbed ones to counter these latter and restore emotional balance. Further, with the increasing number of madhouses in the seventeenth and eighteenth centuries, confinement itself became another aspect of *management* in the view of many, with alleged gains from thus introducing control where matters were out of control and from thus separating the patient from allegedly pathogenic environmental factors. And educational activities, various forms of work, and efforts toward resocialization, all came to be elements in the *management* of insane patients. Then, in his *Traité ... sur ... la Manie* in 1801, Pinel introduced the terms *traitement moral* and *régime moral* for these various aspects of the care of the insane; and in 1806 his English translator, David Daniel Davis, translated these as *moral treatment* and *moral management*.[93] This use of 'moral', of course, did not merely reflect concerns with morality, but, rather, indicated what would today be termed 'psychological' as distinct from 'physical' or 'somatic'.

Of particular note in Pargeter's views on *management* was his emphasis on 'catching the eye' of the insane person in the interest of achieving an 'ascendancy' over him or her.[94] This technique entailed catching and holding the patient's gaze and attention with a complex set of purposes in mind, not all of which seemed to be operative in every case. It served to establish rapport and engender co-operation. It served to calm an excited and overwrought, even maniacal, person. And, at times, it was clearly an interpersonal skill conceived of as bringing mad persons under control in a non-physical manner and without the use of medications, as thus causing them to be more amenable to other aspects of their care, and as leading to their resumption of the self-control that was thought to be associated with a sane state of mind. Pargeter urged that

> practitioners ... before they have recourse to so hazardous an undertaking, should bestow every method in their power to inform themselves of every particular relative to the disorder, and the case in hand ... what may be the probable *remote* cause of the complaint, etc.[95]

He emphasized the significance of the physician having the patient's 'good opinion; a circumstance I always value as a very great point'.[96] He observed that there was a need for 'long experience, and frequent and attentive observation'; that the physician 'must employ every moment of his time by mildness or menaces, as circumstances direct, to gain an ascendancy over them, and to obtain their favour and prepossession'; and that

> he should be well acquainted with the *pathology* of the disease – should possess great acumen – a discerning and penetrating eye – much humanity and courtesy – an even disposition, and command of temper. He may be obliged at one moment, according to the exigency of the case, to be placid and accommodating in his manners, and the next, angry and absolute.[97]

This technique of 'catching the eye' has been more commonly associated with the name of Francis Willis, senior, the physician and clergyman who attended George III in his time of madness in 1788 and 1789. Although his use of it was taken note of by an anonymous author in 1796 who had visited his hospital within the previous year, Willis never wrote about it himself, and so Pargeter appears to have been the first to have published an account of this technique.[98] As is the case with the *moral treatment* that evolved from it, a more detailed examination of the *management* of the eighteenth century soon raises serious reservations about those who maintain that it was primarily controlling and repressive, as well as about anyone who might suggest that all was kindness and humanitarianism. Merely by examining the eighteenth-century selections in Hunter and Macalpine[99] one can see that there were more than a few who emphasized a humane, respectful, and kindly approach in the care of the mad, and the occasional modern scholar has effectively argued the same point.[100] This is not to suggest that abuses did not occur, nor to ignore the implications of the cries for reform and the efforts to that end; and this is not to take anything away from the Retreat at York or from Philippe Pinel. But those turn-of-the-century contributors to improved care for the insane built on an emerging tradition that Pargeter was well aware of, and was personally convinced about on the basis of his own experience.

In several further ways Pargeter reflected transitions that were under way, and gave evidence of them in his *Observations*. He inveighed against the abusive conditions in some madhouses, although he was rather sanguine about public institutions and about those private madhouses that were managed by physicians or clergymen. His criticisms were directed particularly at laymen of questionable qualifications who 'set themselves up keepers of *private mad-houses*'. He asserted that 'it is sufficient to rouse the hearts of Britons, to excite and expedite an enquiry into these enormities, with a spirit proportioned to the atrocity of them'; and, quoting from a publication of the day, he stated that 'a very strict eye should be kept on these *gaolers of the mind*; for if they do not find a patient mad, their oppressive tyranny soon makes him so'.[101] He was concerned that some still countenanced 'beating ... in treating the insane', declaring that 'such usage is on no occasion necessary, self-defence only accepted' and that, if '*management*' failed, '*beating*' would never succeed.[102] He was critical of the frequent tendency to use '*chains* and *cords*' in 'cases of maniacal refractoriness', but he would permit the use of 'a strait-waistcoat' in such instances.[103]

In summary, by the 1790s important changes were under way in the care of mad persons, and Pargeter's *Observations* provides both evidence of several facets of that evolving process, and indicates that he was a participant in it. Within this *management* tradition that was to become *moral treatment*, there clearly were indications that

Introduction by Stanley W. Jackson

control of the disturbed patient, of someone out of control, was thought to be in order. That insane persons might need confinement, control, or even coercion, in the interest of bringing them back to sanity, was a recurrent theme. Yet there were, with significant frequency, indications that kindness was in order, that humanitarian motives prevailed, and that humane treatment was considered crucial in the regaining of a person's sanity.

Notes

1. Roy Porter's (1987) *Mind-Forg'd Manacles. A History of Madness in England from the Restoration to the Regency*, London: Athlone Press, has much to say in this regard for the British scene.

2. William Pargeter (1972) *Observations on Maniacal Disorders* (Reading: for the author). Hereafter this work will be referred to as *Observations*.

3. William Ll. Parry-Jones (1972) *The Trade in Lunacy: A Study of Private Madhouses in England in the Eighteenth and Nineteenth Centuries*, London: Routledge & Kegan Paul.

4. Ida Macalpine and Richard Hunter (1969) *George III and the Mad-Business*, London: Allen Lane, The Penguin Press.

5. Denis Leigh (1961) has stated that Pargeter's unusual career and the astuteness of his book 'suggests that he himself had been the subject of a psychiatric illness', but I have been unable to locate any evidence that would confirm such an inference: *The Historical Development of British Psychiatry: Volume 1, 18th and 19th Centuries*, Oxford: Pergamon Press, pp. 63–4.

6. Richard A. Hunter and Ida Macalpine (1956) 'The Reverend William Pargeter M.A., M.D. (1760–1810)', *St. Bart.'s Hosp. J.*, 60: 56.

7. William Pargeter (1793) *Theoretisch-praktische Abhandlung über den Wahnsinn*, Leipzig: Junius.

8. Ph. Pinel (1806) *A Treatise on Insanity*, D.D. Davis, (trans.), Sheffield: Cadell & Davies.

9. J. C. Heinroth (1818) *Textbook of Disturbances of Mental Life: Or Disturbances of the Soul and Their Treatment*, J. Schmorak, (trans.) and intro. George Mora (1975), 2 vols, Baltimore: Johns Hopkins University Press, 1: 76–7. Also taken note of in 2: 286–7, 305, 308–9.

10. J.B. Friedreich (1830) *Versuch einer Literärgeschichte der Pathologie und Therapie der psychischen Krankheiten: Von den ältesten Zeiten bis zum neunzehnten Jahrhundert*, Würzburg: Carl Strecker,

pp. 502–8. Friedreich (1836) also mentioned Pargeter's work briefly in his *Historisch-kritische Darstellung der Theorien über das Wesen und den Sitz der psychischen Krankheiten*, Leipzig: Otto Wigand, pp. 228–9.

11. Ernst von Feuchtersleben (1845) *The Principles of Medical Psychology* ... , H. Evans Lloyd (trans.), rev. by B.G. Babington (ed.) (1847), London: Sydenham Society, pp. 359–60; D. H. Tuke (1882) *Chapters in the History of the Insane in the British Isles*, London: Kegan Paul & Trench, pp. 142, 512–13; Tuke (1892) *A Dictionary of Psychological Medicine...*, 2 vols, Philadelphia: P Blakiston & Son, 1:24.

12. Throughout this biographical section I am indebted to Hunter and Macalpine, 'The Reverend William Pargeter, M.A., M.D. (1760–1810)'. Their assiduous labours unearthed what little is known about the life of Dr Pargeter.

13. Richard Hunter and Ida Macalpine (1965) 'William Pargeter and the Medical Society of Oxford 1780–3', *Med. Hist.*, 9, 181–3.

14. Ibid., p. 181.

15. [Anon.] (1795) *Formulae Medicamentorum Selectae*, London. See Hunter and Macalpine, 'Medical Society of Oxford', p. 181.

16. It is interesting to note that an earlier physician with a St Bartholomew connection and a significant contributor to medical psychology had also left medicine for the Church. Timothie Bright (?1550–1615) was physician to the hospital and the author (1586) of *A Treatise of Melancholie*, London: Thomas Vautrollier.

17. [Anon.] (1801) *A Sermon, preached in the Protestant Chapel in La Valetta, in the isle of Malta, on Sunday Succeeding the Funeral of Sir Ralph Abercromby, K.B. Commander in Chief of his Britannic Majesty's Forces in the Mediterranean, etc.* Hunter and Macalpine, in 'The Reverend William Pargeter, M.A., M.D. (1760–1810)', p. 55 (fn.), indicate that a handwritten note in the British Museum copy of this 12-page pamphlet says that it was 'Printed in Malta and given by the author William Pargeter M.D. Chaplain to the Garrison, to R. Loder'.

18. Hunter and Macalpine, 'The Reverend William Pargeter, M.A., M.D. (1760–1810)', pp. 54–5.

19. For a detailed study of these matters, see Stanley W. Jackson (1986) *Melancholia and Depression: From Hippocratic Times to Modern Times*, New Haven: Yale University Press, ch. 10.

20. Caelius Aurelianus, *On Acute Diseases and on Chronic Diseases*, I.E. Drabkin (ed. and trans.) (1950), Chicago: University of Chicago Press, pp. 535–59.

21. Aretaeus, *The Extant Works of Aretaeus, The Cappadocian*, Francis Adams (ed. and trans.) (1856), London: Sydenham Society, pp. 301–4.
22. Ibid., p. 301.
23. Galen, *Opera Omnia*, C.G. Kuhn (ed.) (1821–33), 20 vols, Leipzig: Cnobloch, 7: 202; 14: 740.
24. For further detail on these humoral themes, see Jackson, op. cit. (note 19), ch. 10.
25. Thomas Willis, *Two Discourses Concerning the Soul of Brutes ...*, S. Pordage (trans.) (1683), London: Thomas Dring, Ch. Harper & John Leigh, p. 188.
26. Ibid., pp. 188, 201, 205.
27. Ibid., p. 201.
28. Ibid., pp. 201–8. Stygian water meant a caustic or corrosive water. Willis had previously indicated that 'the *Stygian* Waters' were 'distilled out of *Nitre, Vitriol, Antimony, Arsnick, Verdigriece*, and the like' (ibid., p. 189). On analogy to such waters, he thought of the animal spirits in mania as being in rapid and perpetual motion, as corrosive, and as penetrating far and wide in the nervous system.
29. Ibid., p. 188.
30. [Hermann Boerhaave], (1735) *Boerhaave's Aphorisms: Concerning the Knowledge and Cure of Diseases*, London: W. & J. Innys, pp. 323–4.
31. For an account of this process, see Jackson, op. cit. (note 19), ch. 11.
32. Stanley W. Jackson (1983) 'Melancholia and Mechanical Explanation in Eighteenth-Century Medicine', *J. Hist. Med. & Allied Sci.*, 38, 298–319.
33. [Boerhaave], op. cit. (note 30), p. 324.
34. Ibid., p. 313.
35. Ibid., p. 323.
36. Ibid., pp. 324–5.
37. For example, Robert James (1743–5) *A Medicinal Dictionary ...*, 3 vols, London: T. Osborne, 2: *mania*; R. Brookes (1765) *The General Practice of Physic ...*, 5th edn, 2 vols, London: J. Newberry, 2: 138.
38. William Cullen (1785) *Synopsis Nosologiae Methodicae ...*, 4th edn, 2 vols, Edinburgh: William Creech & J. Murray, pp. 257–63; William Cullen (1793) *A Synopsis of Methodical Nosology ...*, 4th edn, corrected and much enlarged, Henry Wilkins (trans.), Philadelphia: Parry Hall, pp. 120–4.
39. William Cullen (1806) *First Lines of the Practice of Physic*, 2 vols in 1, John Rotheram (ed.) New York: E. Duycknick, pp. 485, 492–3.
40. Ibid., p. 497.
41. Ibid., p. 486
42. Cullen, *A Synopsis*, op. cit. (note 38), p. 123.

43. Cullen, *First Lines*, op. cit. (note 39), p. 486

44. Ibid., p. 485

45. Ibid., pp. 485–6.

46. William Cullen (1785) *Institutions of Medicine. Part 1. Physiology*, 3rd edn, Edinburgh: Charles Elliot, pp. 29–32, 62–9, 73–4.

47. William Cullen (1827) *The Works of William Cullen, M.D.* ..., John Thomson (ed.), 2 vols, Edinburgh: William Blackwood, 1: 17; William Cullen (1768–9) *Lectures upon the Institutions of Medicine*, 5 vols, unpublished manuscript of lectures delivered in Edinburgh, located in Yale University Medical Historical Library, 2: 236–43, 245–54, 277–87.

48. Ibid., Lectures, 2: 2–5; Cullen, *Institutions*, op. cit. (note 46), pp. 97–101.

49. Cullen, *First Lines*, op. cit. (note 39), pp. 480–2.

50. Ibid., p. 486.

51. See pp. xx–xxi of this Introduction for an outline of these views.

52. Pargeter, *Observations*, op. cit. (note 2), pp. 6–8.

53. Ibid., pp. 8–9.

54. Ibid., pp. 42–3.

55. Pargeter, *Observations*, op. cit. (note 2), pp. 5–6. This eighteenth-century usage had its roots in Thomas Willis's differentiation of melancholia into a *universal* type *(Melancholia universalis)* and a *particular* type *(Melancholia particularis)*. Thomas Willis (1672) *De Anima Brutorum* ..., Oxford: Ric. Davis, p. 455; Willis (1693) *Soul of Brutes*, p. 188. See also Stanley W. Jackson (1983) 'Melancholia and Partial Insanity', *J. Hist. Behav. Sci.*, 19, 173–84.

56. Pargeter, *Observations*, op. cit. (note 2), p. 6.

57. Ibid., pp. 38–42.

58. Ibid., p. 60.

59. Ibid., pp. 9–10.

60. Ibid., pp. 14–15.

61. Ibid., pp. 16–26.

62. Ibid., pp. 26–7.

63. Ibid., pp. 29–38.

64. Ibid., p. 29. For a detailed account of degeneration, see Georges Genil-Perrin (1913) *Histoire des origines et de l'évolution de l'idée de dégénérescence en médecine mentale*, Paris: A. Leclerc; for a useful capsule account, see Erwin H. Ackerknecht (1959) *A Short History of Psychiatry*, Sulammith Wolff (trans.), New York: Hafner, ch. 7.

65. Jackson, *Melancholia and Depression*, op. cit. (note 19), pp. 328–39. Regarding Methodism in particular, see Leigh, op. cit. (note 5), *British Psychiatry*, p. 66 and Michael MacDonald (1981) 'Insanity

and the Realities of History in Early Modern England', *Psychol. Med.*, 11: 11–25.

66. William Buchan (1813) *Domestic Medicine* ..., new, correct edition, enlarged – from the author's last revisal, Boston: Joseph Bumstead, p. 289. This mention was present in the first edition, published in Edinburgh in 1769, and continued in the subsequent editions.

67. Pargeter, *Observations*, op. cit. (note 2), p. 10.

68. W. Griesinger (1867) *Mental Pathology and Therapeutics*, 2nd edn, C. Lockhart Robertson and James Rutherford, (trans), London: New Sydenham Society, pp. 1, 3, 7, 9.

69. Pargeter, *Observations*, op. cit. (note 2), pp. 12–14

70. Ibid., pp. 62–93.

71. Ibid., pp. 95–108.

72. Ibid., pp. 104–8.

73. Ibid., p. 62.

74. Ibid., p. vi.

75. This was John Monro (1715–91), the second of the Monros to be associated with Bethlehem Hospital. His *Remarks on Dr. Battie's Treatise on Madness* will be discussed in the following section ('Moral management and moral treatment').

76. Nathaniel Wanley (1634–80) was a clergyman who authored (1678) *The Wonders of the Little World: Or, a General History of Man* ..., London: T. Basset, R. Cheswel, J. Wright & T. Sawbridge, from which the case was drawn. Pargeter noted that '*Wanlye*' in turn had taken this case 'from *Heywood*, in his *History of Angels*'. This referred to Thomas Heywood (*c.* 1574–1641), the English dramatist and poet, and his (1635) *The Hierarchie of the Blessed Angells* ..., London: Adam Islip.

77. Levinus Lemnius (1505–68), a Dutch physician who later became a clergyman, wrote about the temperaments, the diseases to which they were thought to be prone, and remedies for those diseases in *The Touchstone of Complexions* ..., Thomas Newton (trans.), London: Thomas Marsh, 1576. Originally published in Latin in 1561, this work was frequently drawn upon by Robert Burton in *The Anatomy of Melancholy*.

78. In pre-Homeric times, according to Greek legend, the three daughters of Proetus were driven mad by an offended deity. They were said to have either slighted the worship of Dionysus or presumed their beauty to be equal to that of Hera. They wandered about 'with all manner of unseemliness', including the delusion that they were cows. Melampus was reputed to have been the first mortal to practise medicine and to possess

prophetic powers. Called upon to help Proetus' daughters, he cured them by drastic purging with hellebore. It has been said that he was the discoverer of hellebore.

79. Jean Baptiste van Helmont (1579–1644), the Flemish physician, whose restatement of the chemical philosophy was to be particularly influential in the emerging medical chemistry of the seventeenth century.

80. This referred to the familiar Biblical account of Saul, the first king of Israel, whose melancholic illness was cured by the music of David's harp (Samuel I: 16), and whose experience has been so often cited in references to music as treatment for mental disorders.

81. William Perfect (1737–1809), an English surgeon who came to concentrate his professional efforts on working with mad persons, owned a private madhouse, Malling Place, at West Malling, Kent. The case cited by Pargeter was described as part of Case XIV in Perfect's (1787) *Selected Cases ... of Insanity, Lunacy, or Madness ...*, Rochester: W. Gillman, an extensive collection of case histories that had two earlier editions and several later editions under various titles.

82. Of Swiss-French origins, MD from Bologna, and associated with Geneva, Théophile Bonet (1620–89) is best known for his extensive compilation of post-mortem cases that made a significant contribution to the emerging field of pathological anatomy. The case described by Pargeter was taken from Bonet's (1683) *Mercurius compitalitius ...*, Geneva: Leonard Chouët, Lib. XI, Mania, case XI, where Bonet indicated that he in turn had taken this case report from Jean Denis (d. 1704), a French physician who was at the centre of both experimentation and controversy regarding the transfusion of blood in Paris of 1667–8 (*Lettre écrite à Monsieur *** par J. Denis ... touchant une folie invétérée qui a esté guérie depuis peu par la Transfusion du Sang*, Paris: J. Cusson, 1668).

83. Richard Mead (1673–1754), perhaps the most eminent English physician of his time and well known abroad, was a friend of Isaac Newton and a staunch advocate of the application of Newtonian thought in physiological and medical explanations. The cases cited are to be found in *The Medical Works of Richard Mead, M.D.*, London: C. Hitch *et al.*, 1762, pp. 486–8.

84. Pargeter, *Observations*, op. cit. (note 2), p. 49.

85. Ibid., pp. 61–2.

86. Ibid., pp. 50–3, 57–61.
87. William Battie (1758) *A Treatise on Madness*, London: J. Whiston & B. White, p. 68.
88. John Monro (1758) *Remarks on Dr. Battie's Treatise on Madness*, London: John Clarke.
89. Ibid., pp. 35–6.
90. Ibid., p. 37.
91. Ibid., p. 40.
92. On another topic, he cites the works of both Battie and Monro from which I have just quoted (see Pargeter, *Observations*, op. cit. (note 2), p. 115).
93. Ph. Pinel (1801) *Traité Médico-Philosophique sur L'Aliénation Mentale, ou La Manie*, Paris: Richard, Caille & Ravier; Pinel (1806) *Treatise on Insanity*, op. cit. (note 8). Joseph Daquin (1733–1815), an older contemporary of Pinel, who assumed responsibility for insane patients in the hospital at Chambéry in 1787, published *La Philosophie de la Folie* in 1791, a work that was informed by humanitarian ways and values akin to those of Pinel. He employed the term '*traitement moral*', and emphasized the importance of 'les secours moraux' in the treatment of the mad. Unable to locate a copy of the first edition of *La Philosophie de la Folie* in North America, I have been limited to the use of the second edition published in 1804. By 1804 Daquin had come to know of Pinel's work, was familiar with *Traité* ... *sur* ... *la Manie*, had revised his own book in ways influenced by Pinel, and had dedicated his second edition to Pinel. It seems likely to me that Daquin only introduced the term '*traitement moral*' in his second edition, but he had already emphasized the importance of 'les secours moraux' in his first edition (and used the term in his sub-title); and his orientation provides one more indication of eighteenth-century trends in the care of the mad. Joseph Daquin (1804) *La Philosophie de la Folie*, 2nd edn, Chambéry: P. Cleaz.
94. Pargeter, *Observations*, op. cit. (note 2), pp. 49–53, 57–61.
95. Ibid., pp. 61–2.
96. Ibid., pp. 59–60.
97. Ibid., pp. 49–50.
98. [Anon.] (1796) *Détails sur l'établissement du docteur Willis, pour la guérison des Aliénés*, in *Bibliothèque Britannique, Littérature*, Geneva. Cited by Richard Hunter and Ida Macalpine (1963) *Three Hundred Years of Psychiatry, 1535–1860*, London: Oxford University Press, pp. 538–9. It is

of interest to note here that, just a few years earlier, another technique for psychologically influencing sufferers in the interest of therapeutic gain, of one mind influencing another, had won both fame and notoriety in Paris. But, although the holding of the patient's gaze might be said to be a common feature, Franz Anton Mesmer's (1734–1815) technique was very different – he used magnets, and he made physical contact with his patients, sitting in front of them with their knees touching his, pressing their thumbs in his hands, looking fixedly into their eyes, touching their hypochondria, and making passes with his hands over their limbs. His explanations were also very different – he energetically opposed any psychological explanation for his results, naming his approach *animal magnetism* and attributing the effects to a *magnetic fluid* akin to the imponderable fluids of contemporary physical science. And there is no evidence that his technique was known to either Pargeter or Willis (Henri F. Ellenberger (1970) *The Discovery of the Unconscious: The History and Evolution of Dynamic Psychiatry*, New York: Basic Books, pp. 57–69).

99. Hunter and Macalpine, *Three Hundred Years of Psychiatry*, op. cit. (note 98).
100. Alexander Walk (1954), 'Some Aspects of "Moral Treatment" of the Insane up to 1854', *J. Ment. Sci.*, 100: 807–37; Roy Porter (1981–2) 'Was There a Moral Therapy in Eighteenth Century Psychiatry?', *Lychnos*, pp. 12–26.
101. Pargeter, *Observations*, op. cit. (note 2), pp. 123–9.
102. Ibid., pp. 129–31. In the eighteenth century, that such physical mistreatment of insane patients was often rumoured, was likely enough if one can judge from Cullen's countenancing of it in his advice on the care of the mad, and was occasionally documented as in the case of George III. For Cullen, see Cullen, *First Lines*, op. cit. (note 39), p. 488. For George III, see quotation from Countess Harcourt in Kathleen Jones (1955) *Lunacy, Law, and Conscience 1744–1845: The Social History of the Care of the Insane*, London: Routledge & Kegan Paul, pp. 41–2. For further mention, see Macalpine & Hunter, *George III and the Mad-Business*, op. cit. (note 4); Parry-Jones, *Trade in Lunacy*, op. cit. (note 3).
103. Pargeter, *Observations*, op. cit. (note 2), pp. 131–2.

OBSERVATIONS

ON

MANIACAL DISORDERS.

OBSERVATIONS

ON

MANIACAL DISORDERS.

By WILLIAM PARGETER, M.D.

Orandum eft, ut fit mens fana in corpore fano.

Juv.

READING:

PRINTED FOR THE AUTHOR, AND SOLD BY SMART AND
COWSLADE, READING; J. MURRAY, FLEET-STREET,
LONDON; AND J. FLETCHER, OXFORD.

M DCC XCII.

PREFACE.

TO form juſt notions and draw fair concluſions on any ſubject, it is thought neceſſary, by *ſome* writers, that the ſtricteſt attention be paid to ſyſtematic order and method, in the arrangement of ideas, and the conduct of arguments : but on a ſubject ſo abſtruſe and intricate as the preſent, it is impoſſible to adhere to rules, even if I were inclined to ſubſcribe to the above opinion.

I have not ventured to eſtabliſh a theory of my own on this occaſion, but have adopted Dr. *Cullen's* idea, and likewiſe his terms of *excitement* and *collapſe* : in doing this, I feel no heſitation; becauſe he not only comes nearer to a right theory of this diſorder than any former writer, but I do not think it poſſible for human underſtanding to advance any other. And for my own

infor-

information on this head, I am obliged to the library of a phyfician of fingular eminence—Lord *Litchfield's* Clinical Profeffor.

Of the authors whofe fentiments I have adopted, fome I have mentioned, and others I could not call to my recollection.

I have not fpoken to all the *genera* of the difeafe, according to the nomenclature, or the claffification of nofologifts; becaufe there are feveral that I never met with in practice, confequently it cannot be fuppofed that I fhould be able to ftate them. I have omitted other remarks, becaufe they are too common and obvious. The *definition* of madnefs, by the confent of all writers, is delirium *without* fever : and here I cannot forbear an attempt to fettle a point, concerning which, moft people have been too hafty in forming their opinions. Some few years ago, a cafe in medicine occurred, which agitated this kingdom, and engaged the attention of all *Europe.* This cafe was univerfally, I believe, thought to have been *maniacal*; and left this idea fhould be a future reproach to us from other nations, I firmly deny the pofition in the following fyllogifm :

Quid eft infanitas ?
Infanitas eft, delirium *fine* febre—
Etat ægro febris——ergo,
Æger non erat infanus.

It is impoffible to draw a right conclufion from falfe premifes. And if the premifes in the above fyllogifm are not true, the fyftem of *nofology* is entirely fubverted.

In

In reciting the cafes, I have forborne to mention the names and refidences of the patients, becaufe I would not, on any confideration, wound their own feelings, or thofe of their friends; and if any fhould imagine themfelves alluded to, I beg to affure them, that on my part, it is not with the leaft intention of being pointed or offenfive.

The few *formulæ medicamentorum* introduced, are meant barely as a guide to young practitioners, to be regulated as circumftances may require.

Should the enfuing obfervations be favourably received, I may probably, at fome future time, purfue the fubject to a greater extent; but if not, I fhall never again obtrude myfelf on the notice of the public.

E R R A T A.

PAGE. LINE.

31   18   For *Infanity was manifeftly the caufe of religious delufion*, read *religious delufion was manifeftly the caufe of Infanity.*

52   18   For *cachexcy*, read *cachexy.*

58   18   For *in confequence of having had an unfortunate parturition*, read *in confequence of an unfavourable parturition.*

75   6   For *fubftracting*, read *fubtracting.*

100   6   For *inferiore*, read *inferiora.*

Other inaccuracies, it is hoped, will be excufed.

OBSERVATIONS

ON

Maniacal Diforders.

————————

THE fummit of luxury to which the prefent
age has attained, muft naturally tend to inter-
rupt the regularity of the animal economy, and
to enfeeble the generations of men.   But the
improvements which the practice of medicine
and the enquiry into the ftructure of the human
frame have received of late years, afford a
ftrong prefumption, that difeafe has arrived at
the height of its dominion, and that mankind

may

may at length regain the energy and longevity of their anceftors. It muft, however, be acknowledged, that the hideous malady which fo amazingly prevails at this day, fhould feem to denote, that we have made no very confiderable advances towards the recovery of our ancient vigour: and it muft excite a refleCtion as humiliating to the pride of fcience, as painful to the feelings of philanthropy, that in the courfe of almoft three thoufand years no medicines have been difcovered on which any reliance can be placed.

It would be almoft too fhocking to portray the real features of this terrible complaint; yet, in order to a conception of it, they ought in fome meafure to be contemplated. Let us then figure to ourfelves the fituation of a fellow creature deftitute of the guidance of that governing principle, reafon—which chiefly diftinguifhes us from the inferior animals around us, and gives us a ftriking fuperiority over the beafts that perifh. View man deprived of that noble endowment, and fee in how melancholy a pofture he appears. He retains indeed the

outward

outward figure of the human fpecies, but like the ruins of a once magnificent edifice, it only ferves to remind us of his former dignity, and fills us with gloomy reflections for the lofs of it. Within, all is confufed and deranged, every look and expreffion teftifies internal anarchy and diforder. The wretched victim now triumphs in imaginary pleafures, and is now tortured with ideal woes—his diftempered fancy transforms his beft friends into the bittereft enemies, and he views them with implacable averfion or with difdain—he fwells with pomp, or fhrinks with terror, fometimes breathing menaces againft his oppofers, and fometimes trembling with apprehenfions of their difpleafure. He now relapfes into fullen infenfibility —the delirium again returns, and he raves with all the vehemence of exafperated fury—far from attending to his own prefervation, he is incapable of ufing the leaft effort for his fafety —reduced to the mental weaknefs of a child, he is indebted to the friendly care and precaution of others for his very exiftence. Without this neceffary interpofition, the wretched fufferer

would

would but too frequently execute deliberate vengeance on himfelf, and thus end his miferies and his life together. What then can be more melancholy—what misfortune more afflictive, than to labour under the preffure of this dreadful malady?

The frequency of this difeafe renders it truly alarming—it fhould therefore be one of the firft objects of the phyfician's meditation and refearch; and though it has been treated of by many authors of note, it muft be acknowledged that their compofitions betray much confufion and contradiction—and it may be fufpected, that in practice, by too generally attending to appearances, and overlooking the caufes, phyficians have, with a pardonable but hafty zeal to do every thing, fometimes done much harm.

The *Nofologifts* of the prefent era are far from being confiftent in their arrangement of the feveral *genera* of this difeafe. *Profeffor Cullen* in his *Nofology of Mania,* has with the greateft propriety altered the arrangement of the two *genera Mania et Melancholia,* which

Linæus

Linæus and others have adopted, and comprehends his idea of the complaint in two words—*Infania Univerfalis.*——Synop. Nos. Method. G. LXVII.

The doctrine of *Mania* includes in fome degree that of *Melancholia*, confequently they cannot be *generically* different. *Melancholia* often arifes to fo high a degree as nearly to be confounded with *Mania.* The learned *Dodonæus* obferves well, by faying " *Madnefs* and *Melancholy* are fo nearly allied, that oftentimes *Madnefs* turns to *Melancholy*, and frequently the beginning of *Melancholy* affumes the appearance of *Madnefs.*" The diftinction is fo difficult, that if I was to attempt it, you would probably apply to me the words of *Parmeno* in the *Eunuch:*

> Incerta hæc fi tu poftules
> Ratione certa facere, nihilo plus agas,
> Quam fi des operam, ut cum ratione infanies.
>
> TER. EUN. ACT I. SC. I.

Practical writers have generally diftinguifhed *Mania* by the *fury, impetuofity,* and *angry temper*

per attending it—but such a complaint may take place without any impetuosity. The term *furibunda*, which *Linæus* has admitted into his character of *Mania*, should be left out, because I have often seen *Maniacs*, who at different times were *furious* and *peaceful*, without any remission of the essential characteristic symptoms of the disorder *Infania Univerfalis*—but in lower degrees of *Melancholia*, the error of the intellectual power is confined principally, often entirely to one subject.

The *Profeffor* takes notice of *two ftates* of the *brain*; the one he terms *excitement*—the other *collapfe*. *Collapfe* may be defined a morbid diminution of the tone of the brain, and of the motion of the nervous fluid. The term *excitement* must be obvious to every one. I am inclined to be of opinion, that *collapfe* or undue *excitement*, takes place, more or less, in every species of *Mania*. It is manifestly perceptible, from the confideration of the ftates of found sleep and dreaming, that different parts of the brain, or different faculties of the intellect, can be in different degrees of *excitement* at the same
time

time. The delirium occurring at falling afleep, or at firft waking out of fleep, fhews, that the perfect exercife of our intellectual faculties requires fome *equality* in the *excitement* of every part of the brain; and the delirium in the inftances above mentioned, feems to depend on an *unequal excitement* of the different parts. To apply thefe propofitions to our prefent purpofe, we may obferve, that fometimes a *collapfe* of one part of the brain interrupts the communication of the due *excitement* of the whole, and thus induces delirium. Any excefs, efpecially a partial excefs of *excitement* will have the fame effect; for the regular order and fucceffion of *ideas*, with which judgement is immediately connected, depends upon a certain degree or meafure in the force and velocity with which thefe *ideas* take place, and therefore it is, that every caufe of hurry throws us into confufion, which is a momentary and flight degree of *Mania*. Every fudden emotion is liable to have this effect, and fome emotions produce it more permanently. Thus we fhew that an *uncommonly encreafed excitement* of the

brain,

brain, is a principal circumſtance in *Mania*—a poſition which I think is confirmed by the increaſed impetus of the blood, a common cauſe of too great *excitement* of the brain inducing *delirium* in *phrenitis*, and fever; for the *delirium* occuring in theſe caſes, can only be explained upon this principle. To put it beyond all doubt, we may obſerve, that in moſt inſtances of *Mania*, in every inſtance of the *Mania furibunda*, a violently *encreaſed excitement* is manifeſt from the increaſe of ſtrength and vigour which takes place; of which have been ſeen many wonderful inſtances, even in females, before weak and delicate. Another proof of this poſition is, that *Maniacs* reſiſt all thoſe *ſeaative* powers which in natural health are ſo remarkable for inducing ſleep. They ſuſtain watching for an almoſt incredible length of time. Another proof may be deduced from their inſenſibility to the power of cold; they feel no bad effects from its impreſſions; they reſiſt indeed impreſſions of every kind: this perhaps may be no proof of an *excited* ſtate of the brain. They reſiſt alſo, for

the

the moſt part, the power of opium, and thoſe
anodynes which render the nervous power im-
movable by ordinary impreſſions. It has been
alledged, that every tone of the mind has a ſtate
of the body correſponding with it; if it is the
caſe, I think the *fury* of *Maniacs* is a mark of
a ſtrongly *excited ſtate* of the mind, and therefore of the brain: the ſame takes place in the
paroxyſms of anger, which is *furor brevis*.
The *Mania furibunda* depends more manifeſtly
upon a greater *excitement*, probably affecting
every part of the brain. In the *Mania tranquilla*, probably a great degree of *collapſe* affects
one part of the brain, while other parts are
unuſually *excited*, or even the common degrees
of *excitement* remains in theſe: for an *inequality*
of the *excitement* of the brain will diſturb the
exerciſe of the intellectual functions, as much
as a violent *increaſe* of it—but the phenomena
attending this ſtate will not be ſo evident as
dreadful.

We are acquainted with many of the *proximate cauſes* of *Mania*; but whether they ope-

rate

rate directly by inducing *collapse*, or by bringing
on an *increased excitement*, is not determined.
The principal of these are, *various topical affections of the brain—watry effusions—obscure
schirri—preternatural ossifications—*and *numerous causes of increased impetus of the blood in
the head.* Many cases of *Mania* are short and
transitory, and admit of very sudden changes
—these certainly are not dependant on any *organic* affection—others continue through life;
it is equally improbable, that any *organic* affection is here present: many are cured, and
frequently relapse; this gives us some suspicion
of a peculiar affection of the brain; but we are
not clear concerning the nature of this state.
There must indeed be in every case of *Mania*,
in all probability, some peculiar corporeal morbid state, with which that peculiar state of the
mind is connected; and it is more than probable, that the corporeal part affected is the
brain.

It may therefore be proper, before we proceed
to the consideration of the *remote causes* of

Mania,

Mania, to inveftigate the ftate of the brain, which at that time takes place. The fum of all the obfervations made before *Boerhaave*'s time, by diffections, are given in his *Aphorifm,* 1121, " And we muft take notice, that by anatomical infpection it has been made evident, that the brain of thofe is *dry, hard, friable,* and *yellow* in its cortex ; but the veffels *turgid, varicous,* and diftended with *black* and very *tough blood*." *Morgagni* in his *Epift. Anat. Med. de Mania,* &c. fpeaking of the ftate of the brain, in feveral cafes where he had an opportunity of obferving that ftate, defcribes it in one cafe in thefe words, " But nothing occurred which was more worthy of obfervation, than the *hardnefs* of the cerebrum ; for whether we cut into its medullary or cortical fubftance, the fubftance appeared to be *very hard,* at the fame time that the fubftance of the cerebellum, or at leaft the cortical part of it, was even rather *fofter* than ufual."—In another cafe, he has thefe words, " Although I found water extravafated under the *pia mater,* yet the cerebrum was of fuch a *firmnefs,* that I then never remembered

C 2   to

to have diffected one fo *hard*." *Dr. Hunter*
found the principal parts of the medullary fubftance of the brain in *Idiots* and *Madmen*, fuch
as the *thalami nervorum opticorum*, and *medulla
oblongata* to be entirely changed from a medullary to an *hard, tough, dark-coloured* fubftance,
fometimes refembling white leather. Moft of
the *anatomifts* feem to confider the *preternatural
hardnefs* of the cerebrum and cerebellum, as
the only circumftance that deferved particular
notice in the brains of the *Maniacal* patients
they had diffected. But *Valfalva*, who has but
one cafe, obferved on opening the fkull, fome
little white bodies at the fides of the longitudi-
nal finus in the dura mater externally; fome of
which were round, others long, and fome of a
figure irregular, but all of a *foft* confiftence;
and he thought that they had their origin from
a concreted humour, becaufe he had feen fimilar bodies from concretions of *pus*, ftagnating
about the fame membrane, in patients who
had died from wounds of the head—but in
that finus was a flender polypous concretion,
which extended itfelf through the whole length
of

of the cavity. The brain was *moiſt*, and in its
larger ventricles was a little quantity of ferum :
—however, in the plexus choroides, pretty
large glandular bodies appeared prominent,
which had been *indurated* into a *ſolid, yellow*,
and fomewhat globular body. And *Dr. Sim-
mons*, phyſician to St. Luke's Hoſpital, in ſix
caſes out of a great many more that he had an
opportunity of diſſecting, remarks, that he found
a confiderable *ferous*, or *watry effuſion*, not only
within the ventricles, but likewiſe between the
pia mater and the furface of the brain; and
ſuſpects that ſuch an *effuſion* frequently takes
place in *inſane* patients, and confiders it as a
circumſtance likely to prove of confiderable
importance in the *Pathology* of *Mania*. I
have had but three opportunities myſelf of inveſ-
tigating the ſtate of the brain of patients who died
maniacal— the brain appeared in all three caſes,
more *flabby* than ufual ; and in one caſe, the
pineal gland was furrounded with a *watry fluid*,
and was almoſt obliterated. After all, I am
of opinion, that no true judgment can be formed

from any morbid appearances which the brain may exhibit on diffection, becaufe it will be impoffible to determine whether thofe appearances are *caufes* or *effects*. Suppofe a cafe of infinity from fome known caufe, and another utterly unaccountable, and the appearances on diffection the fame, it may naturally be prefumed that they are *effects*. But fuppofe that two men lofe their reafon by repeated intoxication, and the fame appearances fhould be difcovered on diffection, we fhall feel no hefitation in pronouncing them *caufes*—but fhould the brain of thefe men betray different appearances, it would be difficult to determine whether fuch appearances are *caufes* or *effects*, and this uncertainty muft prove a bar to the furtherance of *pathological* knowledge of mental derangement.

The *original* or *primary* caufe of Madnefs is a myftery, and utterly inexplicable by human reafon. Thus far, however, has been difcovered, that there is a fluid continually fecreted by the cerebrum and cerebellum, and propelled

into

into the nervous tubuli, from whence it is called a nervous fluid, &c This fluid (or electric aura, as some style it) is capable of manifold variations—either in its quantity, it may become too much or too little—or it may admit of many alterations in its quality, and may become thicker or thinner in its consistence than it ought to be—it may likewise, from causes to us unknown, assume other and different qualities. A certain morbid or *irritating* principle or quality of that fluid acting upon the brain is the *primary* cause of Infanity, with all the unaccountable phenomena which attend it; but what the *specific* nature of that morbid quality or principle is, it is impossible to conceive, and it will, no doubt, for ever remain a secret.

——Nec meus audet
Rem tentare pudor, quam vires ferre recusent.

Here our researches must stop, and we must declare, that " wonderful are the works of the Lord, and his ways past finding out."

Of

Of the ordinary *remote* caufes, we may enu-
merate the following: Firft, thofe acting on the
mind; as fudden and violent emotions, or paffions. *Fear* has often been productive of permanent Madnefs. It is a very common expreffion to fay, *fuch a man was frightened out of his
wits.* Great and habitual fear is attended with
an unufual wafte or depreffion of the nervous
power, whence a lefs vivid and generous circulation, and thence a diminifhed perfpiration.

―Ubi vehementi magis eft commota *Metu* mens
Confentire animam totam per membra videmus :
Sudores itaque, et pallorem exiftere toto
Corpore, et infringi linguam vocemque aboriri :
Caligare oculos, fonere aures, fuccidere artus.
Denique concidere ex animi terrore videmus
Sæpè homines : facilè ut quivis hinc nofcere poffit,
Effe animam cum animo conjunctam; que cum animi vi
Percuffa eft, exin corpus propellit et icit.

                            LUCRET.

The operations of the mind on the body, and *é
contra*, is alfo a myftery, and does not come under
a mechanical mode of reafoning ; it being impoffible to decypher and trace out the feveral
                                  fteps

fteps and ways of procedure of thofe agents, which can by no means be brought under the cognizance of our fenfes. In inquiries therefore of this kind, there muft be allowed fome further *data* than need be, in fuch as are merely *phyfical. Baron Haller,* in his firft lines of Phyfiology, obferves, that " they have behaved modeftly, who confefling themfelves ignorant, as to the manner in which the body and mind are united, have contented themfelves with proceeding no farther than the known laws, which the Creator himfelf has prefcribed; without inventing and fupplying us with conjectures not fupported by experience." *Anger*—fudden anger or refentment, acts, with fome perfons, in one circumftance, fimilar to fear; all the blood veffels of the extremities and fuperficies of the body are contracted, pallidnefs and trembling are induced, and the diftribution thus rendered unequal blood is accumulated about the heart and head.

" There,

" There is a paffion, whofe tempeftuous fway
Tears up each virtue planted in the breaft.
For *pale and trembling* anger rufhes in,
With *fault'ring fpeech*, and *eyes* that *wildly flare·*"

ARMSTRONG.

Joy, the fweet banifher of care, if it be fud‑
den and exceffive, fo impairs the vital powers,
that Infanity, or immediate death is fometimes
the confequence. An excefs of *joy* or *fudden
furprife*, might render the fentient principle
inattentive to the accumulation of blood in
the right ventricle of the heart; whence no
fyftole enfuing, a fatal collapfion of the pulmo‑
nary arteries and the lungs might enfue, and the
circulation inftantaneoufly ftop. Neither is it
very ftrange on proper reflection, that great and
fudden alterations in the mind fhould act as
fatally as great and fudden alterations in the
air, and more inftantaneoufly; their operation
immediately affecting thofe tender and intimate
receffes, and that exquifite *medium* or fluid,
which may primarily, however inconceivably,
conftitute the *nexus*, or union of life with matter.

All

All the ſtrong and durable depreſſing paſſions—
Grief, ſadneſs, deſpair; and thus we explain the
common effect of great misfortunes; great re-
verſes in the purſuit of *wealth* or *ambition*; in
ſhort, all diſappointments of *keen deſires.*—To
this head therefore, we refer the *Erotomania,*
i. e. Deſiderium *Amantium* pudicum. LINNÆI
Gen. Morb. lxxxii.——That great maſter of
allegorical fiction, *Spencer*, leads us to the
dreary manſion of *Deſpair*, in the following
lines, which, as awfully deſcriptive, ſtand un-
rivalled.

" Ere long they come, where that ſame wicked wight
His dwelling has, low in a hollow cave,
Far underneath a craggy cliff ypight,
Dark, doleful, dreary, like a greedy grave,
That ſtill for carrion carcaſes doth crave:
On top whereof ay dwelt the gaſtly owl
Shrieking his baleful note, which ever drave
Far from that haunt all other chearful fowl;
And all about it wand ring ghoſts did wail and howl!
That darkſome cave they enter, where they find,
That curſed man *(Deſpair)* low ſitting on the ground,
Muſing full ſadly in his ſullen mind;
His greaſy locks, long growen, and unbound,

D 2   Diſorder'd

Diforder'd hung about his fhoulders round,
And hid his face; through which his hollow eyne
Look'd deadly dull, and ftared as aftound;
His raw bone cheeks, through penury and pine,
Were fhrunk in o his jaws, as he did never dine.
His garment nought but many ragged clouts,
With thorns together pinn'd and vatched was,
The which his naked fides he wrapt abouts;
And him befide there lay upon the grafs,
A dreary corfe, whofe life away did pafs,
All wallow'd in his own yet luke-warm blood,
That from his wound yet welled frefh alas
In which a rufty knife faft fixed ftood,
And made an open paffage to the gufhing flood!"

Thofe depreffing paffions, by their continuance, keep the folids fo long in a ftate of relaxation, that the orifices of the fecretory glands
lye fo very open and expofed, as to fuffer an
efcape even of that balfamic fluid which is dif-
penfed to the feveral parts of the body for
their nourifhment and fupport; by which means,
the body is robbed of its moft neceffary juices,
which, by their aptitude to cohefion, and the
fmall momentum or force with which they
are brought to the fecretory orifices, as foon as

they

they are propelled through, they ſtick to and lodge upon the ſkin, and occaſion that greaſy clammineſs commonly called, a *cold ſweat*.

Avarice envy, jealouſy, and an habitual indulgence of *pride*, are oftentimes productive of Madneſs. Of *arrogant Inſanity*, the ingenious *Dr. Perfect* relates the following aſtoniſhingly curious caſe:—Some years ago, a poor man, who having ſtudied the art of government and the balance of the European power with greater attention than his buſineſs, grew inſane, and fancied himſelf a king, and, in this ſituation, was admitted into the orkhouſe of St. Giles's in the Fields, where there happened to be an idiot of nearly his own age; this imaginary king appointed the idiot his prime miniſter, beſides which poſt, he officiated as his barber and menial ſervant; he brought their common food, and ſtood behind his majeſty whilſt he dined, when he had permiſſion to make his own repaſt. There would ſit, the king upon an eminence, and his miniſter below him, for whole days, iſſuing their precepts to their ima-

ginary

ginary fubjects; in this manner they lived about
fix years, when, unfortunately, the minifter, im-
pelled by hunger, fo far deviated from his line
of allegiance, as to eat his breakfaft before his
fovereign appeared, which fo exafperated the
king, that he flew upon him, and would certainly have put a period to his exiftence, if he
had not been prevented; when his anger was
thought to have abated, the minifter was again
introduced to his quondam fovereign, but he
feized him immediately, and could never after
be prevailed on to fee him. The degraded
minifter catched a fever in his exile, and when
his majefty was beginning to relent, and almoft
prevailed upon to forgive him, he died; which
had fuch an effect upon this fancied monarch,
that, after living almoft without fuftenance, in
a continued filence, a few weeks, he died of
mere grief. Ill-fated monarch! thou couldeft
not, as can the illuftrious monarch of the prefent day, if his minifter were to " pay his tri-
bute into the treafury to which we muft all be
taxed," appoint another, who would guide the
reins of empire with as much prudence and

fuccefs

ſucceſs as the preſent one hath done: throughout thy whole territory, there was not found
one hardy enough to engage in the arduous taſk;
and equally unable to ſupport the weight of
government alone, as to deſcend to the peaceable, but unhonoured, vale of retirement, thou
didſt quietly yield up thy life and ſceptre together! Perhaps it may afford ſome ſatisfaction
to the reader, to be informed, that this anecdote
is founded in fact; the name of the king having
ſtood in the books of the pariſh, with the addition of " the lunatic king," for ſeveral years,
the firſt entry being January 1ſt, 1727.

Intenſe ſtudy and *application of mind*, is one
of the moſt common cauſes of Madneſs, eſpe-
cially if this application is directed to one object, or to objects of a ſimilar nature. When the
mind is inceſſantly engaged in the contemplation of one object, only one part of the *ſenſo-
rium* is acted upon, and that is always upon
the ſtretch; it is not relieved by the action of
the other parts, and therefore is ſooner fatigued
and injured. If one, or only a ſmall number

of

of mufcles is continually kept in motion, the body fuffers more than if the fame quantity of action was fucceffively divided among all the mufcles: it is the fame with the brain; when its different parts act alternately, it is not fo foon weary; the part at reft recovers itfelf, while the others are exercifed: this change from labour to reft, is the fureft method of preferving the organ. *Meditation* alfo, by keep-ing the nerves too long in a ftate of action, waftes the fpirits too much, and hinders the brain from preparing them; fo that this impor-tant fluid, the moft highly prepared in the hu-man body, and which is moft neceffary for the performance of its functions, is either deficient, or undergoes fome alterations, which muft ine-vitably produce many diforders. *M. Pafcal,* a man of an uncommonly ftrong mind, did fo much injury to his brain by *intenfe application* and *deep thought,* that he always imagined there was a gulph of fire near him; the conftant agitation of fome of his fibres conveyed this fenfation to him perpetually; and his reafon, fubdued by his nerves, could never get the

better

better of this idea. *Gaſpar Barloeus*, an orator, poet, and phyſician, was ſenſible of theſe dangers, and often uſed to warn his friend *Hughens* of them; indeed, he wrote the following advice to him : " nec literas, nec verſus reſcribe, ne in novum diſcrimen valetudinem dubiam adducas. Facile enim ex attentione incaleſcent ſpiritus, hinc ſanguis, hinc habitus corporis "—*Barloei Epiſt. lib* 1. *ep.* 4. But he was, notwithſtanding, regardleſs of himſelf, and weakened his brain ſo much by exceſſive ſtudy, that he thought his body was made of butter: in this perſuaſion, he carefully avoided coming near the fire; till at laſt, wearied with continual apprehenſions, he threw himſelf into a well. I have read of a man who was employed day and night in reading, reflecting, and making experiments; he firſt loſt his ſleep, then was ſeized with ſome tranſitory fits of lunacy, and at length became quite mad. *Wepfer* relates of a young man who having inceſſantly applied himſelf to his ſtudy both day and night, fell into a delirium, which ſoon degenerated into madneſs, in a fit of which he wounded ſeveral perſons, and at

E   length

length killed his keeper.—*Obſervat de Affect.*
capit. obſ. 8 5, *p.* 327.   But without going any
further for inſtances, a young man, a ſtudent
at an academy at *Berne,* having taken it into
his head that he could diſcover the quadra-
ture of the circle, died mad at the *Hotel Dieu*
of *Paris.*   Our Philoſophical Tranſactions and
the phyſiological parts of many foreign literary
Emphemerides furniſh us with numerous ex-
amples of the morbid or fatal effects of *exceſ-*
five ſtudy. As the humours are more abundant-
ly derived to any part which is in action, there
muſt be a greater accumulation in the brain
of the ſtudious, which increaſing the tone and
motion of veſſels, produces many fatal diſ-
tempers.—The *remote* cauſes already enumerated, are ſuch as act upon the mind.

Secondly, thoſe whoſe firſt operation is on
the body—as *poiſons,* chiefly of the intoxi-
cating kind. By *opium,* we often produce temporary delirium, and by employing it in larger
doſes, we might occaſion a more permanent
Madneſs. It is but too often the conſequence

of

of *intoxication*, from the too liberal, or too frequently repeated ufe of other inebriating fub-
ftances.   Ill managed, and long continued
courfes of *mercurial medicines* have produced this
diforder.   It has alfo been known to originate
from the ufe of pomatum, in which fome *mercurial* preparation was an ingredient; this is the
practice of fome hair-dreffers, with the idea of
deftroying animalcula, but it is highly injurious
and abominable; and fo likewife is that of
mixing quick lime with their powder.   It has
fometimes been imputed to *fuppreffed evacuations* and *repelled eruptions*; the firft, and perhaps the fecond of thefe caufes may be fufpected
to act by caufing a determination of blood to
the brain.   I knew a lady who was very much
troubled with an eryfipelas in the face, to remedy which, fhe imprudently had recourfe to
the external application of *vitriolated argill*
(or alum) *whey*, and in confequence became
mad.   In whatever way we may interpret
the effect, a *turgefcence of the feminal veffels*—
an high degree of *luft* and *falacity*, have induced
Mania.   How thefe caufes operate or are fitted

to produce either an *excefs* of *excitement* or *col-lapfe*, or *inequalities* in thefe ftates, I fhall not attempt to explain: it is fufficient, that the facts are really true.

When we behold the moft fhining charac-ters—our relations—our deareft friends and companions, whofe reafon lies either " buried in the body's grave," or who linger out an haplefs exiftence in a rueful ftate of idiotifm or fatuity, we cannot but be affected with the moft lively fenfations of pity and regret. Under the influence of paffions and reflections, which occurrences of this nature are apt to excite, we are fometimes undutifully inclined to withdraw from Providence that veneration and refpect which it claims from all; as if it were poffible for Heaven to be deficient in integrity of defign —wifdom of appointment, or uniformity of con-duct. But why fhould we *charge God foolifhly*, with what is generally occafioned by an unrea-fonable indulgence of our fenfual appetites, or a too fervile compliance with the prevailing manners.

But

But to be more particular :—To thefe *remote* caufes which have been enumerated others may be affigned as *auxiliaries* in fpreading the unhappy difeafe And firft, the *Luxury* of the times. Our anceftors deviated from the regular and temperate manner of life—our grandfathers were therefore weaker than our anceftors, were more delicately and effeminately brought up, and their offspring were ftill weaker than themfelves; and we of the fourth generation, have fcarcely any ideas except what we learn from hiftory, of former health and vigour. Thefe remarks bear confiderable analogy to that moral and fatyrical climax in *Horace :*

> " Ætas parentum, pejor, avis tulit
> Nos nequiores, mox daturos
> Progeniem vitiofiorem."

But befides this degeneracy, which we thus derive from our progenitors, we may add, that by the frequent and immoderate ufe of tea— long fafting—inflammatory food—turning day into night, and night into day, the order of

nature

nature is moſt ſhamefully inverted—our time, which was given us for far more valuable pur-poſes, is vilely proſtituted—every active inſtru-ment of health is mutilated and maimed—our bodies become enervated—our intellectual fa-culties impaired, and the date of life abridged; at length we ſink into the arms of everlaſting reſt, with a *faſhionable* death, the natural con-ſequence of a *faſhionable* life. With what additional force muſt the practice and purſuit of the foregoing evils operate on female con-ſtitutions, whoſe frame and contexture are ſo delicate and tender; and it is ſeriouſly to be remarked, that in this age, it is eaſier to meet with a *mad,* than an *healthy* woman of *faſhion.* A deſcant on the preſent mode of living, as it reſpects diet—the non-naturals—the baneful effects of the public education of females, &c. would be in this place a digreſſion, but may probably be conſidered at ſome future period. For the preſent, I ſhall only obſerve, that the grievances above ſtated are inconteſtible, and experience furniſhes us with numerous and enormous inſtances, of the pernicious conſe-
quences

quences of luxurious indulgence to the morals
and conftitutions of mankind.

Secondly, *Fanaticifm* is a very common caufe
of Madnefs. Moft of the Maniacal cafes that
ever came under my obfervation, proceeded
from religious *enthufiafm*; and I have heard it
remarked by an eminent phyfician, that almoft
all the infane patients, which occurred to him
at one of the largeft hofpitals in the *metropolis*,
had been deprived of their reafon, by fuch
ftrange infatuation.   The *doctrines* of the
Methodifts have a greater tendency than thofe
of any other fect, to produce the moft deplorable effects on the human underftanding.
The brain is perplexed in the mazes of myftery, and the imagination overpowered by the
tremendous defcription of future torments.——
I fhall fubjoin a cafe or two, in which Infanity
was manifeftly the caufe of *religious delufion*.

CASE I.

I was fent for to a refpectable farmer,
in the country; I found him very low and
melan-

melancholy—inconfiftent in his converfation, and feemed to labour under great diftrefs concerning his future ftate. His friends had been obliged fome time before to place him in an houfe for the reception of lunatics. I could do him very little fervice, as I was unable to remove the caufe. This man's misfortunes originated in a very curious fact: he was publicly reproved by a clergyman for fleeping during divine fervice, which gave him fo much offence, that he feceded from the Church, and attached himfelf to the *Methodifts*; thefe *deluded people* foon reduced him to the unhappy ftate in which I found him. I could not learn on ftrict enquiry, that previoufly to this circumftance, he had exhibited any fymptoms of mental derangement; but was efteemed a lively, chearful, and pleafant companion.

CASE II.

I was defired to vifit a woman who refided at no great diftance from the man whofe cafe has juft been defcribed. I found her fitting

up

up in the bed—fhe was wrapped about the head, neck and fhoulders with cloaks and flannels—fhe received me with a fmiling countenance, and when I enquired into her complaints, fhe laughed, and enumerated a great variety of fymptoms; but I could not really difcover that fhe had any bodily indifpofition, except what was occafioned by laying in bed. In a chair at the bed-fide, were, *Weftley's Journal, Watts's Hymns, the Pilgrim's Progrefs*, and *the Fiery Furnace of Affliction*. I prefcribed according to the ufual form, but could do her no good; and I was afterwards informed, that fhe became fo mad as to require confinement. I was told by her hufband, that there was not the leaft pre-difpofition to Infanity before this attack, and it appeared that a *Methodift preacher*, who had much infefted the parifh, was frequently in her company, and they were perpetually converfing on religious topics.

I attended a young woman with a peripneumony, occafioned by fome tea, or bread

F   and

and butter paffing down the trachea in a fit
of laughter; as the fymptoms were acute
and fufpicious, I paid more than ordinary attention, vifiting her twice, and often three times
a day. I hardly ever went into the room, but
I faw a man with a book in his hand, who I
afterwards learnt was a *Methodift*. One day
when I called, the girl was exclaiming, " Oh
fweet Chrift! Dear Chrift! I do love Chrift!"
I afked her what fhe meant, and fhe told me
" She had feen, and had been talking with, her
dear Chrift." The patient fortunately loft her
complaint, and being enabled to return to her
former occupation, her mind was gradually
weaned from thofe *delufions*, which might probably have terminated in *confirmed Mania*. The
advantage which this *fanatic* took, of the girl's
ignorance and indifpofition, may very aptly be
compared to the conduct of thofe inhuman
wretches, who avail themfelves of the confufion at a fire, to plunder the fufferers. The
prevalence of *Methodifm*, with its deplorable
effects, in the neighbourhood where this girl

refided,

refided, might be afcribed to an opulent Tanner, who maintained a preacher in the capacity of a domeftic chaplain, a failor in the laft war. He was one day haranging on the fubject of Hell flames, and took occafion to obferve, that he could not give a defcription by any means adequate to the horrors of that place, although he had been there eleven months; a wag, whom curiofity had led to hear him, called out, " I wifh you had ftaid there another month, and then you would have gained a fettlement." Such dreadful infatuation is the more melancholy, as it tends to augment the number of *fuicides* in a nation, which is fuppofed to be more generally addicted to this crime, than any other people in Europe: indeed, the French have adopted our word *fuicide* into their language, as an Anglicifm. Such confequences, however, from this particular caufe, muft convince all perfons of a found underftanding, of the errors of thofe tenets, which caufe, or very greatly conduce to it; fince genuine Chriftianity muft very pow-

erfully

erfully deter men from this unnatural violence.
Whatever a late bishop's charity has disposed
him to suggest, in extenuation of such voluntary
fatalities from despair, and in his not wholly
despairing notions of their eternal state; it is
incontestable that this temerity is an horrid vio-
lation of the strongest instinct, which the Author
of universal Nature has implanted into ours.
Indeed, where this effect arises from indisputa-
ble Insanity, through whatever cause, or previous disease, the guilt will vanish, as the mise-
rable patients in that situation must be merely
passive. It is believed, that some *enthusiastic
preachers* have exulted in these dismal events,
as proofs of their powers of convincing and
converting: but it is really amazing, as I cannot suppose them to be actuated by any malignant intention, that a few catastrophes of their
hearers or penitents being sent to Bedlam or
to the grave, have not effectually convinced
them, that these cannot be the fruits of true
religion; and thence, of the consequent absur-
dity and evil of their conduct. To such indeed

we

we may certainly well apply the obfervation of
a late good and ingenious poet:

> " And when their fins they fet fincerely down,
> The'll find that their religion has been one."

Thirdly, a *Lunatic Anceftry*. When Madnefs exifts in the blood of families, and fhews
itfelf regularly in the feveral branches of the
pedigree, ill concerted alliances will always
keep up the general tendency to the difeafe.
What then fhall be faid of thofe, who either
from ambitious or lucrative motives, ftifle the
feelings of honour and humanity, and fordidly
fubmit to form connections which entail mife_
ries on their pofterity, more grievous than death
itfelf? Such matrimonial contracts, therefore,
fhould be avoided, and, if poffible, prevented
by every one who is a well-wifher to fociety:
indeed, I feel no reluctance whatever, in pronouncing tho e who engage in, and thofe who
encourage and promote fuch alliances, to be, in
the ftricteft fenfe, *enemies to their country*. If
the fymptoms do not immediately appear, but

lie

lie dormant for a time, we are juſtified, I think, in deeming thoſe perſons at leaſt *amentes*, if not abſolutely *maniaci*.

From the doctrine which has been laid down, and the conſequent remarks, it will be neceſ-ſary to propoſe ſome method of cure, as far as it is practicable: and in order to introduce this important object, it will be proper, Firſt, to point out ſome, or moſt of the *diagnoſtic* ſymp-toms, which accompany this diſeaſe; and firſt, thoſe which attend *melancholia,* or as it may be denominated, *Mania tranquilla,* or *innocua :* ſuch as, thoughtfulneſs--profound taciturnity--a fond-neſs for ſolitude—obſtinacy—refuſing all kinds of ſuſtenance, but ſometimes preternaturally voracious—coſtiveneſs—no urine, or little and pale—pulſe ſlow, and frequently imperceptible —watchfulneſs—a fuſco-pallid complexion— flatulency in the præcordia—ſometimes eruc-tations of an acrid-porraceous and bilious hu-mour—they will lament, weep and ſigh heavily,

without

without any apparent caufe—they are fometimes, though very rarely, feen

> " In moody madnefs, laughing wild
> Amid fevereft woe."

This is moft horrible indeed; and thofe who
have once experienced fuch a fpectacle, I am
confident, will never wifh it a fecond time.

Poets have drawn many fine and ftriking
images of *Melancholy*; particularly *Beaumont* and
Fletcher, who reprefent her amidft bats and
owls, in the depth of folitude and gloom.

> " Hence all you vain delights,
> As fhort as are the nights,
> Wherein you fpend your folly;
> There's nought in this life fweet,
> If men were wife to fee't,
> But only *Melancholy*:
> Oh, fweeteft *Melancholy*!
> Welcome folded arms, and fixed eyes,
> A figh, that piercing, mortifies,
> A look that's faftened to the ground,
> A tongue tied up without a found.

Fountain

Fountain heads and pathlefs groves,
Places which pale paffion loves;
Moon-light walks, when all the fowls
Are warmly hous'd, fave bats and owls;
A midnight bell, a parting groan,
Thefe are the founds we feed upon!

The fublime *Milton*, at the opening of his
Il Penferofo, has thefe beautiful lines:

" Hence, vain deluding joys,
The brood of folly, without father bred,
How little you befted,
Or fill the fixed mind with all your toys!
But hail, thou Goddefs, fage and holy!
Whofe faintly vifage is too bright,
To hit the fenfe of human fight;
Come, penfive Nun, devout and pure,
Sober, ftedfaft, and demure,
All in a robe of darkeft grain,
Flowing with majeftic train,
And fable ftole of Cyprufs lawn,
Over thy decent fhoulders drawn.
Come, but keep thy wonted ftate,
With even ftep and mufing gait,
And looks commercing with the fkies,
Thy rapt foul fitting in thine eyes;

There

There held in holy paſſion ſtill,
Forget thyſelf to marble, till
With a ſad leaden downward caſt,
Thou fix them on the earth as faſt."

But nothing can be more poetically deſcriptive of *Low-ſpiritedneſs* or *Melancholy*, than the
ſubjoined inimitable lines from *Cowper's Poems*,
vol. 1.—*Retirement.*

" Look where he comes—in this embower'd alcove
Stand cloſe conceal'd, and ſee a ſtatue move :
Lips buſy and eyes fixt, foot falling ſlow,
Arms hanging idly down, hands claſp'd below,
Interpret to the marking eye diſtreſs,
Such as its ſymptoms can alone expreſs.
That tongue is ſilent now, that ſilent tongue
Could argue once, could jeſt or join the ſong ;
Could give advice could cenſure or commend,
Or charm the ſorrows of a drooping friend.
Renounc'd alike its office and its ſport,
Its briſker and its graver ſtrains fall ſhort :
Both fail beneath a fever's ſecret ſway,
And like a ſummer-brook are paſt away.
This is a ſight for pity to peruſe,
Till ſhe reſemble faintly what ſhe views ;
Till ſympathy contract a kindred pain
Pierc'd with the woes that ſhe laments in vain.

G   This

This, of all the maladies that man infeſt,
Claims moſt compaſſion and receives the leaſt.

——— ———— ————

'Tis not, as heads that never ach ſuppoſe,
Forgery of fancy and a dream of woes :
Man is an harp, whoſe chords elude the ſight,
Each yielding harmony diſpos'd aright.
The ſcrews revers'd (a taſk which if He pleaſe,
God in a moment executes with eaſe)
Ten thouſand, thouſand ſtrings at once go looſe,
Loſt, till He tune them, all their power and uſe.

——— ———— ————

No wounds like thoſe a wounded ſpirit feels,
No cure for ſuch, till God, who makes them, heals."

After theſe ſymptoms have prevailed for a
greater or a leſs time, thoſe which diſtinguiſh
the *Mania furibunda* begin, ſometimes ſud-
denly, and in a moment, to make their appearance. They then become reſtleſs—more lo-
quacious—haughty and ſupercilious in their
demeanour——are ſuſpicious—fickle—captious
and inquiſitive about trifles—have a furious aſ-
pect—redneſs of the eyes—a quick ſenſe of
hearing—are irritable, particularly at meals—
they entertain an inveterate averſion to particu-

lar

lar perfons. As the complaint proceeds to a
more confirmed ftate, there is an almoft conftant and tremulous motion of the eye-lids,
which is extremely characteriftic of the diforder. They will hallow—fwear—pray—fing—
cry—laugh, and talk lafcivioufly, almoft in the
fame inftant. They have an high degree of
falacity—a prodigious degree of ftrength—a
total difregard to cleanlinefs—are malicious and
mifchievous, attempting their own lives, or of
thofe about them. The face exhibits a fhining
or greafy appearance. They are extremely
hypocritical, and oftentimes endeavour to per-
fuade the by-ftanders that they are dead; and
fometimes affect to have loft the ufe of their
limbs. Thefe laft appearances frequently accompany *Hypochondriafis* or *Melancholia.*

Several very curious accounts of mental per-
verfion are recorded by *Zac. Lufit. Prax. ad-
mir.* lib. 1. obf. 44 and 45. *Nic. Tulp.* Obf.
Med. lib. 1. c. 18. *Roderic. Fonfeca de Sanit.
tuend,* c. 24. *Bartholine* Hift. Anat. cent. 1.
hift. 79. *Lemn. de Complex.* l. 2. c. 6. *Tral-*

lian.

lian. l. 1. c. 16. *Zuing Theat.* vol. 1. lib. 1.
p. 8. *Laert.* lib. 2. c. 18. *Cœlius Rhodig.*
Antiq. lib. 1 . c. 2. *Girald.* Hift. Poet dialog.
3. *Reynolds* of the Paffions, chap. 21. p. 213.
I cannot forbear inferting two of the moft remarkable, as they ftrongly illuftrate the preceding remark.

The firft, from *Heywood,* in his *Hiftory of
Angels,* lib. 8. p. 551. taken notice of by *Mr.
Wanlye* in his *Wonders of the Little World,* lib.
2. c. 1. A young man, troubled with an *hypochondriacal* diforder, had a ftrong imagination
that he was dead, and not only abftained from
food, but importuned his parents, that he might
be carried to his grave and buried, before his
body was putrified. By the advice of his phyficians, he was accordingly laid upon a bier,
and carried upon men's fhoulders towards the
church; but upon the way, they were met by
two or three merry fellows, hired for that purpofe, who enquired aloud whofe corpfe they
were going to inter; and being informed by
the bearers, *Well,* fays one of them, *the world*

is

*is happily rid of him, for he was a man of a
wicked life, and his friends have cause to rejoice
that he did not make his exit at the gallows.*
The young man hearing this, raised himself
upon the bier, and told them *he had never deserved the character they gave him, and that if
he was alive, as he was not, he would teach them
to speak better of the dead:* but the fellows continuing to treat him with opprobrious language, being not able to bear it any longer,
he leaped from the bier, fell upon them with
great fury, and beat them till he was quite
weary. This violent agitation gave such a
different turn to the humours of his body, that
he awaked, as one out of sleep or a trance, and
being carried home, and taken proper care of,
in a few days he recovered his former health
and understanding.

The second, from *Lemnius de Complex* lib.
2. c. 6. A person of rank verily believed he
had departed this life; and when his friends
intreated him to eat, or threatened to make
him, he absolutely refused it, telling them that

food

food could be of no fervice to a dead perfon. Having continued in this condition feven days, and his friends fearing that his obftinacy would really prove the occafion of his death, bethought themfelves of the following ftratagem :—They fent into his bed-chamber, which they had purpofely made as dark as poffible, fome fellows wrapped in fhrouds, who carried with them victuals and drink, fat down at the table, and began to eat heartily. The difordered man, feeing this, afked who they were, and what they were about. They replied, they were dead perfons. *What then*, fays the patient, *do the dead eat? Yes, yes*, fay they, *and if you will fit down with us, you may eat likewife.* Upon this, he jumps out of bed, and falls to with the reft; and having made a hearty meal, and drank a compofing draught which they provided for him, he went to bed again, fell into a fine fleep, and in a fhort time recovered his health and fenfes.

Thofe who labour under a fevere degree of this diforder, imagine themfelves to be cattle

of

of particular kinds, and endeavour to imitate their voices; others fancy they are made of a teftaceous fubftance. Some think themfelves kings—prophets; others, a grain of wheat—glafs, or wax. I think *Mr. Pope* has fomewhere defcribed the extravagant reveries of a difordered imagination in the following line:

" Men prove with child as pow'rful fancy works."

There are other phenomena which accompany this difeafe. Mad people are frequently very quick in repartee, and exceedingly acute in their remarks: fome of them have an extraordinary poetic turn, and will recite lines and paffages from various authors, and in different languages, which they could not fo eafily call to memory while the intellects were perfect. On this occafion, we might apply to them what *Shakefpeare* fays in *Hamlet.*

" How pregnant his replies are,
A happinefs that madnefs oft hits on,
To which fanity and reafon could not be
So profperoufly delivered of."

It

It is further worthy of remark, that perfons, who in their found ftate of mind, laboured under an invincible impediment of fpeech, have, when afflicted with this malady, ex-preffed themfelves without the leaft hefitation. Mad people generally live to a great age, and there is often a difpofition to corpulency. Thin perfons, of a dry tenfe fibre, and of a dark melancholic temperament—an hairy and robuft conftitution—of middle age, or rather under —a quick, penetrating, and difcerning genius, *et è contra*, are moft fubject to madnefs.

It is impoffible to form a certain *prognofis* of Mania, while the original caufe is enveloped in fo much obfcurity. Indeed, the *prognoftic* art is at beft, but conjectural; yet in thofe cafes of madnefs which are the effects of the *pathemata animi* or *metaftafes*, the *prognoftic* fymptoms are more eafily diftinguifhed, than when occafioned by *labes hereditaria.* or mor-bid or topical affections of the brain; but as we are never clear when thofe affections do

take

take place, the *prognosis* must always be uncertain.

The chief reliance in the cure of insanity
must be rather on *management* than medicine.

The *government* of maniacs is an art, not to
be acquired without long experience, and frequent and attentive observation   Although it
has been of late years much advanced, it is
still capable of improvement.   As maniacs are
extremely subdolous, the physician's first visit
should be by surprize.   He must employ every
moment of his time by mildness or menaces,
as circumstances direct, to gain an ascendancy
over them, and to obtain their favour and prepossession.   If this opportunity be lost, it will
be difficult, if not impossible, to effect it afterwards; and more especially, if he should betray any signs of timidity.   He should be well
acquainted with the *pathology* of the disease—
should possess great acumen—a discerning and
penetrating eye—much humanity and courtesy
—an even disposition, and command of tem-

H   per.

per. He may be obliged at one moment, according to the exigency of the cafe, to be placid and accommodating in his manners, and the next, angry and abfolute.

I fhall fubjoin three or four cafes, in which *management* feemed to be attended with the moft defirable effects.

CASE I.

When I was a pupil at St. Bartholomew's Hofpital, as my attention was much employed on the fubject of Infanity, I was requefted by one of the fifters of the houfe, to vifit a poor man, an acquaintance of her's, who was difordered in his mind. I went immediately to the houfe, and found the neighbourhood in an uproar. The maniac was locked in a room, raving and exceedingly turbulent. I took two men with me, and learning that he had no offenfive weapons, I planted them at the door, with directions to be filent, and to keep out of fight, unlefs I fhould want their affiftance. I then fuddenly unlocked the door—rufhed

into

into the room and caught his *eye* in an inftant. *The bufinefs was then done*—he became peaceable in a moment—trembled with fear, and was as governable as it was poffible for a furious madman to be.

C A S E II.

A young lady, who refided at a village near the metropolis, had been for fome weeks on a vifit to a friend, at a diftance from home. In a few days after her return, her natural fpirits and vivacity gradually forfook her; fhe became penfive—morofe—fond of being in her own room and alone—fhe would take no nourifhment, unlefs to avoid importunities. After I had informed myfelf particularly refpecting the family—occafional vifitors in her late excurfion, &c. I was introduced to her room, and found her in a thoughtful pofture, her elbow on the table, and refting her cheek upon her hand. She did not, for fome time, feem to know that any body was in the room; at length fhe looked up, and the moment I caught her *eye*, for, till then I had been filent, I told her I was perfectly

fe&ly acquainted with the caufe of her complaint, and converfed with her on thofe topics,
I thought moft fuitable to her cafe, and at laft
perfuaded her to come down to dinner with the
reft of the family, and to drink two or three
glaffes of wine, and to join in the converfation
of the table. I recommended an immediate
change of refidence—gave directions refpecting
diet—-exercife-—amufements—reading—converfation—and had foon the pleafing fatis-
faction to be informed of the lady's perfect
recovery.

It may be proper to remark that a thorough
knowledge of the *pathology* was abfolutely neceffary in this cafe. The patient had taken emetics with the fetid and deobftruent gums, and
antifpofmodics, under a fuppofition that fhe laboured uuder a cachexcy. When, therefore, phyficians who have not made infanity their ftudy,
meet with low, nervous, or *hypochondriacal*
cafes, they fhould immediately propofe a con-
fultation with one who has. By fuch feafon-
able interpofition, the principles of the difeafe

may

may be fuppreffed on their firft appearance, and evils of the moft dreadful nature prevented.

This branch of my fubject furnifhes me with an opportunity which I cannot refift, of offering a few remarks on a matter, which is well entitled to confideration. It but too often occurs, in this faithlefs and degenerate age, that we obferve men fteal on the confidence and efteem of fufceptible females, by the beguiling arts of flattery; and by converfation, arrayed in the fhape of reciprocal affection. Having, at length, by thefe wiles, effected a conqueft over their inclinations, they are perfidioufly and ungeneroufly forfaken; and the fenfibility of females to focial endearment is fo lively, that there is no pang equal to the forrow of defertion; and the depreffing paffions having once taken poffeffion of their delicate frame, the intellectual faculties are eafily overfet, and thus the unfortunate victim, by fuch difhonourable and barbarous treatment, is torn from the fond embraces of her difconfolate parents and relations—alienated from the fociety of
a wide

a wide and infulted circle of friends and connections—and her mifery increafes, till fhe be-
comes the inhabitant of a mad-houfe, where
fhe paffes the days of beauty, innocence, and
youth, amidft defpair and wretchednefs, till
welcome

> " Death ends her woes,
> And the kind grave fhuts up the mournful fcene."

If the laws of the land have no provifion
againft the increafe of this foreft of all human
violations—if there is no fcourge for fuch
accumulated inhumanity and injury, where
then is the natural fuccedaneum? Where! but
in the arm of vengeance, and the bofom of
bravery? And yet are we not forbidden to
abftain from blood, on any provocation?
We are, and we fhould be: a moment's reflection convinces us that the inhibition is
founded in the law of eternal rectitude. It is
man's to err, and to mend; be it God's to pu-
nifh, and to pardon. It is aftonifhing to me,
how fo much villainy can exift in human nature. It is a crime, if poffible, more atrocious
than

than murder; becaufe death is preferable to madnefs. If the modefty of their fex—their fragil and nice contexture, cannot entitle them to our help and defence; furely their fplendid and inimitable virtues—the brilliancy of their genius—their little foftneffes and engaging manners—their counfel and confolation in the hours of affliction and doubt, muft challenge our veneration, excite our regard, and call forth our honour to fofter and protect them. What man can then

"Behold her lying in her cell,
  Her unregarded locks
Matted like *furies* treffes; her poor limbs
Chained to the ground; and 'ftead of thofe delights,
Which happy lovers tafte, her keeper's ftripes,
A bed of ftraw, and a coarfe wooden difh
Of wretched fuftenance."

The man, therefore, who thus wantonly fports with their feelings, and contributes to produce the abovementioned difafters, muft have an heart of adamant—muft be arrived at the higheft pitch of depravity, and ought to be worried from fociety. And I have no-where

met

met with an idea fo precifely equal to the horror with which fuch a truly wicked character
fhould be confidered, as the fentiment of this
couplet.

" Which if in HELL no other pains there were,
Makes one fear HELL, becaufe HE muft be there."

Before I difmifs this point, it may not be
improper to adduce an ancient and hiftorical
fact or two. *Antiochus*, the fon of *Seleucus*,
would have funk under the weight of his diforder, had not the penetration of the attentive
Erafiftratus, his phyfician, difcovered that he
was pining away through love of the fair *Stra-
tonice.—Plutarch. in Demetrio.* And the father of Phyfic could not have faved *Perdiccas*,
King of the *Macedonians*, had he not found
that his diforder, which by every one elfe, was
deemed a confumption, proceeded from an excefs of paffion for the lovely *Phylas*, one of his
father's concubines: " Ex cujus confpectu illum prorfus immutari animadvertit et regem
fanitati reftituit."—*Soranus in vita Hippocrat.*

CASE

C A S E III.

I was defired to vifit a young man. Before I was introduced to the patient, I made fome enquiry about him; and was told, that he had been for feveral days and nights on the bed with his cloaths on, nor would he be prevailed upon to take them off—that he was pe: v'fh— obftinate—refufed all fuftenance—was fil nt, and his face very red. From this reprefentation, I was fearful that his complaint was making a rapid progrefs towards *Mania turibunda.* After fome deliberation, I defired to fee the patient alone—that no one was to co ne into the room till I ftamped with my foot, and then two women were immediately to come up, and to place themfelves one on each fide the bed, and to begin to undrefs him without faying a word. I entered the chamber, and planted myfelf in a direction that I might catch his *eye.* This was not eafy to be done; I, therefore, as I faw occafion, changed my pofition, at which he feemed greatly embarraffed, though not a word paffed on either fide : be

H   ing

ing at length obliged to look up, I *fet* him in
an inftant. Finding that we perfectly underftood each other, I made the fignal, the women
appeared, and executed their orders without
the leaft obftruction. Thus was accomplifhed
in a few minutes what could not be effected
for feveral days and nights. Before I left him,
he quietly drank a bafon of tea, and eat fome
toaft and butter; he was then bled, and took
fome cooling phyfic, which unlocked the fecretory organs, and I had the pleafure, a few
days afterwards, to congratulate him on his
compleat reftoration.

This was a ftrong cafe, and I am convinced,
that if violent means had been ufed, the difeafe
would have appeared in all its fury.

C A S E IV.

A lady became infane, in confequence of
having had an unfortunate parturition. In a
few days, from her derangement, I was defired
to vifit her, and was much pleafed to be informed, that fhe was not apprized of my coming.

ing. Before I was introduced, I underftood
fhe had, from her firft feizure, been fo exceedingly turbulent, as to require coertion. After
fome further enquiries, I begged to fee her
alone: I went fuddenly into the room, and had
her *eye* in a moment. She perfifted in the
fame romantic way of talking, as before I faw
her; but we did not lofe fight of each other
the whole time, neither had I as yet uttered a
fyllable: a fignal which was previoufly agreed
on, being given, the attendants entered, obferving a profound filence, according to my orders,
and began to releafe her, which they foon effected without the leaft refiftance, and immediately withdrew. Being convinced that fhe
was afraid of me, I offered her my hand, which
fhe accepted, and after an hearty fhake, as a
token of amity and peace, I drew a chair, and
in fome meafure relaxing the feverity of my
afpect and demeanour, I endeavoured to draw
her into a more rational converfation; but I
could not accomplifh this by any artifice whatever. However, I could plainly perceive that
I poffeffed, in a confiderable degree, her good

opinion;

opinion ; a circumftance I always value as a very great point, and therefore determined to feize every poffible advantage by it I accordingly prefcribed fome aperient phyfic, which her habit of body rendered her much in need of, and gave it her myfelf, and fhe took it very peaceably. I left her in this ftate for the prefent, nor could I for feveral days gain any advancement in the cure, till the procefs of lactation (the fuppreffion of which caufed her indifpofition) commenced, and then fhe recovered as rapidly as that procefs was completed.

I have to obferve in this cafe, that by *management*, *Mania furibunda* was evidently and happily reduced to *Mania tranquilla*. Before I faw her, fhe had not only beat, and otherwife ill-treated the fervants, but rejected, with fury and difdain, both medicine and food ; by which refractory conduct, her friends were obliged to impofe on her the abovementioned reftraint: but after my firft introduction, fhe took whatever was offered her, without betraying the leaft oppofition. And I am thoroughly convinced,

vinced, that *management* principally contributed
in reftoring a very valuable woman to the en-
joyment of her family and friends.

I have recited thefe cafes out of fome few
others, lefs interefting, barely to demonftrate
what advantages may be accomplifhed by the
art of *management*. The conduct of maniacs to fuperficial obfervers, appears extremely
daring and courageous ; but in reality, they are
exceedingly timorous, and are found to be eafily
terrified And although in the whole courfe
of my practice, I declare, I never failed in re-
ducing them to order, where I made the experiment; yet I muft at the fame time remark,
that there are fome cafes, wherein they are
totally indomable, and where it would be labour in vain, and extremely dangerous even to
attempt it. Practitioners, therefore, before they
have recourfe to fo hazardous an undertaking,
fhould beftow every method in their power to
inform themfelves of every particular relative
to the diforder, and the cafe in hand: as for
inftance, whether there have been any previous
attempts

attempts to fubdue them—what may be the probable *remote* caufe of the complaint, &c. And I fhall conclude this part of the fubject, by noting, that when the art of *management* fails, it will prove equally unpleafant and un-promifing.

When a phyfician has gained this important point, (I mean the art of *management*) he will be greatly affifted in the employment of other remedies. As *Mania furibunda* manifeftly de-pends on an undue and encreafed *excitement*, it fhould be the firft object to diminifh that *excite-ment*, to relax the fyftem, and to derive the blood from the brain; therefore *abftinence* to a very confiderable degree will be proper. Ma-niacs can abftain from food with wonderful perfeverance. The *Stahlians* would, and perhaps properly, confider this as a natural indication: patients in this complaint have lived a confider-able time without any folid food, only em-ploying diluents, fometimes water alone, with-out any diminution of their ftrength.

Bleeding

Bleeding—-wonderfully mitigates morbid heat—proves highly antifpafmodic—leffens the tone of the *fibræ motrices*, and tends to prevent any topical determination. Whenever there is an evident congeftion about the membranes of the cranium and brain, copious and repeated bleedings in the jugular vein will be the moft advifeable.

Arteriotomy in the temples, for this affection of the head, has the authority of phyficians, both ancient and modern; but the turbulence of the patient, in that violent y *excited* ftate, renders that operation, in general, extremely difficult; and, at all times, hazardous.

Phyficians fhould be particularly careful in making a diftinction between the two different temperaments—the *fanguine* and the *melancholic*—as each may require different treatment. Whenever *melancholia* or *mania tranquilla* prevails, and the patient is fullenly intent upon one object, *bleeding* is, in general, of no fervice; though, in fome particular cafes, it may fucceed.

fucceed. In the *fanguine* temperament, on the
other hand, and whenever there is a turgefcence of the arterial fyftem, *venefection*, in
the flighteft ftages of mania, is proper, efpecially if it be complicated with *epilepfia* and
hyfteria, which frequently depend on a plctho-
ric ftate of the fyftem. In cafes of violently
encreafed *excitement*, practitioners have carried
this excefs even *ad deliquium,* with a view to
intercept or fufpend the operations of the mind.
This practice would be judicious if patients
did not bear the lofs of blood fo long as they
do without fainting, and provided there was
no danger of *amentia*, which is a more dreadful fpecies of the diforder; and, when produced by fuch means, is feldom, or ever to be
relieved.

Cupping—with or without fcarification, according to circumftances, may be advifeable in
this complaint.

The *pulfe* is little to be depended on, as it
will be confiderably influenced, if the patient
be fenfible, by emotions, proceeding either
from

from hope or fear. The phyſician ſhould therefore wait ſome time with the patient, till the mind be compoſed, and the pulſe has re-covered its former ſtate, before he attempts to form any judgment from it. It may be ob-ſerved too, that after meals, the pulſations en-creaſe to about ten or twelve in a minute. The pulſe is very fallacious in obeſe habits, from the large quantity of cellular membrane ſurround-ing the arteries. If we judge of the pulſe alike in all conſtitutions, we may be guilty of errors from many circumſtances: from the na-ture of the particular artery, and its different ſituation. If it be deep, though the pulſe be full and ſtrong, it will appear to be weak. If there be many branches running along the radius, beſide that which is generally felt, touching one of *theſe*, which is of a different ſize, inſtead of thoſe which are more diſtinct, will lead into an error.——Again, as ſome branches run over the radius, they may give an hard or ſtronger pulſe than really exiſts. In inflammations it ſometimes occurs that the

K   artery

artery in one arm is more affected than that in
the other; and therefore both arms fhould
always be felt.

Cathartics.———*Cathartics* may be confidered
as evacuants, or as operating by revulfion : in
either view, they muft be regarded as ufeful
remedies in this complaint. As a general evacuant, *purging* is moft proper in the *fanguine*
temperament, and if there is an encreafed determination to the head, it may be doubly ufeful in acting by revulfion. In the *melancholic*
temperament, there is an accumulation of blood
in the venous fyftem, efpecially in the *vena*
portarum, and therefore *purgatives* are particularly indicated ; hence it appears, that in both
cafes, thefe medicines muft be of infinite fervice : but phyficians have differed widely in
the manner of exhibiting them. The ancients
were partial to *acrid purgatives*, efpecially the
black hellebore, and they have fome imitators
among the moderns. This is the foundation of
the praifes beftowed by the ancients on the
hellebore of *Anticyra*, an ifland in the *Archi-*
pelago,

pelago, near *Oeta* in *Theſſaly,* famous for the quantity of *black hellebore* which it produced. *Naviga ad Anticyram* was an indirect inſinuation, that perſons to whom the words were addreſſed, were mad; and *Horace* ſays, lib. 2. ſat. 3. l. 77.

" Audire, atque togam jubeo componere, quiſquis
Ambitione malâ, aut argenti pallet amore;
Quiſquis luxuriâ, triſtive ſuperſtitione,
Aut alio mentis morbo calet: hùc propriùs me,
Dum doceo inſanire omnes, vos ordine adite.
Danda eſt *Ellebori* multo pars maxima avaris:
Neſcio an *Anticyram* ratio illis deſtinet omnom."

And again, l. 165.

" Verùm ambitioſus et audax.
Naviget Anticyram."

——" Tribus *Anticyris* caput inſanabile."—*Perſ.*

Galen de atra bile, *Pliny* and *Dioſcorides* mention a famous cure performed with *black hellebore* by the ſhepherd *Melampus,* upon the daughters of *Prætus,* who were ſo very mad as to fancy themſelves cows. This is the firſt

inſtance

inftance in hiftory, of the exhibition of a ca-
thartic. This medicine feems to promife the
greateft advantages where ftimulating and deobftruent purgatives are chiefly indicated, as in
the *melancholic* temperament, *et Mania a men-
ftruis retentis.* The fubjoined formula, fome-
thing fimilar to that made ufe of by Sir *Clifton
Wintringham,* and as he fays with fuccefs, may
ferve as the bafis of a purgative draught, to be
taken and repeated as circumftances may direct.

      ℞ Rad. hellebori nigri.
         Tart. folub. ā ʒij.
         Fol. fenæ ℥fs. decoque cum aq. diftillat.
         ℔j. ad colatur. ℥x.

      ℞ Hujus clari liquoris ʒx.
         Pulv. &c. m. f. hauftus.

The *tinctura hellebori* may likewife be employed with the fame view, from ten drops to
a dram, or upwards, as the cafe may require.
In *obftructed catamenia,* this medicine received
unbounded encomia from Dr. *Mead,* who fays,
" Ex omnibus autem, quæ menfes movent
maximè, fingularem virtutem habere depre-
hendi

hendi *helleborum nigrum*; ita ut illum vix un-
quam fpem fefelliffe meminerim. Idcirco *tinc-
turæ melampodii* cochleare minimum ex aquæ
tepefactæ hauftulo bis die affumi jubeo. Et illud quidem notabile obfervavi; quod quoties
cunque aut propter malam partium conforma-
tionem, aut alia quacunque de caufa, fine ef-
fectu datum effet hoc medicamentum, fanguis
per alias vias propulfus fuerit: unde clariffime
conftat, quanta vi fanguinem propellendi pol-
leat ifta medicina. ' The Doctor's extravagant
commendation of this *emenagogue* has not however been juftified by fubfequent experience.
In *Mania*, occafioned by *fuppreffed hæmorrhoids*, acrid *purgatives* of the *aloetic* clafs, will
often fucceed in bringing them on again. With
this intention, the following pills may be given
in large and repeated dofes.

R Aloes focot. ℈ij.
Pulv. ipecac. gr. iv m. f. pil mediocres.

But as maniacs are extremely fubject to
coftive bowels, *cooling aperients*, conftantly employed, fo as to keep the body open, are, for
the

the moſt part, to be preferred; becauſe by the
mildneſs of their operation, they occaſion little
diſturbance to the ſyſtem, and as the *neutral
ſaline laxatives* do not produce the reſtringent
effects which are common to the acrid and
heating purges, they are entitled to the firſt
conſideration. The *tartarum ſolubile* has been
generally preſcribed as an *eccoprotic*, particularly adapted to this complaint. The following may ſerve as a ſpecimen for a draught, to
be taken and repeated according to its effects.

R Decoct. hord. ten. ʒxiv.
  Tart. ſolub. ʒij plus vèl minus.
  Syr. roſæ ʒij m. f. hauſtus.

The *phoſphorated ſoda*, introduced as a medicine by Dr. *George Pearſon*, is an elegant neutral ſalt, and is reported to have this advantage
over moſt of the ſaline *purgatives*, that it is
not ſo unpleaſant to the palate, having much
the ſame flavour as common ſalt when diſſolved
in broth or gruel; and as it does not occaſion
cholicky or griping pains, it is well ſuited to
weak

weak bowels. From fix drams to an ounce, or more, may be given for a dofe.

Emetics. The ancients in *Madnefs,* as well as in many other diforders, as we are informed by *Celfus,* in the 13th chapter of his fecond book, ufed *emetics* of the *draftic* clafs, particularly *veratrum,* or *white hellebore.* Their catalogue of *emetics* was very defective, and the few they were acquainted with, were either extremely rough and unfavourable in their operation, or too gentle and ineffectual. *Hippocrates* underftood the method of moderating the force of *vomits,* but others lefs fkilful, were often deceived. The *veratrum* was fometimes fatal, and the action of others doubtful; but in our times, we employ thofe that are fafer and lefs vehement in their operation, among which we may juftly give the preference to that *American* root *ipecacuanha,* and the *antimonium tartarifatum,* (late *tartar emetic*) both of which are not unfriendly to the nervous fyftem, and may be exhibited with perfect fafety, either conjointly or feperately. But as the ftate of the

ftomach

ftomach in *Mania* is frequently oppofed to fenfibility, it may be moft prudent to adminifter
them together, but it is impoffible to prefcribe
the quantity or proportion of each; they muft
be varied according to the effects.

℞ Vin ipecac. ℥ifs.
  Antimon. tart. gr. ij. m. f. hauft. emet. cum vel
  fine regimine folito fumend. et repetend.
  p. r. n.

vel.

℞ Tart. antimon. gr. ifs.
  Pulv. ipecac. ℈j. m. f. pulvis emet. ut fupra
  fumend.

Emetics may be given with fingular advantage in every degree of defective reafon, from
the *hypochondriafis, Melancholia, et Mania tranquilla,* to the higheft pitch of *Mania furibunda.* The phenomena of this difeafe fhew,
that the fault is principally lodged in the fluids,
and confifts in too great a thicknefs of them,
or a diffipation of the moft volatile moveable
parts. If the digeftive powers are morbidly
affected, the *ingefta* will not be fufficiently
concocted; hence the chyle and the vaporous
                                    halitus

halitus of the blood, the animal fpirits will become vitiated—the abdominal vifcera weakened and obftructed, and their action deftroyed, whilft the blood paffing through different degrees of fpiffitude, at length degenerates into what the ancients called *atra bilis*. Thus congeftion is formed in and about the trunk of the *vena porta*, and the beginning of the *meferiac artery*. Befides the evident ufe of *emetics* in difcharging morbid collections from the ftomach, they alfo, by agitating the whole frame, excite a general commotion in the nervous fyftem—promote an uniform circulation —produce a determination to the furface of the body—reftore a more equal excitement— evacuate ferous accumulations from every cavity in the body, and remove obftructions in the fanguiferous fyftem. They ought always to precede the ufe of other remedies, *bleeding* only excepted.

Fontanels. Difcharges by *iffues* or *fetons* are of the firft importance in all difeafes of the head, and fhould be employed in every fpecies

L   of

of *Mania*, from whatever cause it may proceed.
The practice of making *artificial ulcerations* is
of very antient date. *Setons* were first made
use of by *Columella*, in the reign of *Claudius*,
and their utility is testified by many writers of
note: as, *Galen*, *Platerus*, *Glandorpius*, *Forestus*,
Angelus Sala, *Ambrosæus Paræus*, *Rammazzini*,
Sydenham, *Morton*, *Nicholas Robinson*, Baron
Van Swieten, *Ruyfch*, and Sir *John Pringle*.
Diemerbroek gives them the title of *prestantif-
sima subsidia*—*Hoffman* calls them *egregia pro-
phylactica*. *Willis* in his *Pharmaceutice Rationalis*, edit. *Oxon*, 1675. sect. 3. cap. 4.—*de
fontic. five fontanell.* makes the following remark: Multo certe rectius materiam morbificam
περι τον εγκεφαλον deponi solitam fonticulus in
Brachio anticipat, in crure revellit, et paulo in-
fra caput excitatus, eam inde derivat. Hinc
ad graviores cerebri aut meningum affectus, in-
fantibus, ac pueris, foveam nuchæ incidimus;
adultis, ac senibus cauteria ex utroque spinæ
latere, inter Homoplatas applicamus; ibidem-
que duas fontanellas plurium piforum capaces,
cum magno sæpe commodo procudimus. *Fon-*
tanels

tanels poffefs great power in draining morbid
ferum from the blood, and of courfe wonder-
fully temper the animal fpirits. It is a miftaken
notion, that they induce debility, and weaken
the conftitution; for, on the contrary, they
ftrengthen and invigorate the habit by fubftracting the enervating caufe.

Blifters——Of the modus operandi of *cantharides* on the fyftem, there has been much
controverfy. And although phyficians have,
with a laudable fpirit of enquiry, debated the
fubject with much earneftnefs and ingenuity,
yet on what principles their virtues are founded,
has never been clearly or correctly afcertained.
The Arabian phyficians were the firft who
ufed blifters. They were of opinion, as appears from *Oribafius*, the firft Arabian author,
who mentions them, that they operated by
diffolving the lentor of the blood. *Bellini* and
Baglivi entertained the fame idea: but the ingenious Dr. *Percival*, of *Manchefter*, has fully
refuted that doctrine. However I may be inclined, at a future period, to engage in this

L 2   difpute,

difpute, it certainly is not my province on this occafion. I have only to fpeak of them here as they may or may not be beneficial in a variety of circumftances attending *maniacal* diforders. Many practitioners have recommended the application of *blifters* to the head, and particularly *Suturis Cranii*, *in mania furibunda*: This practice I fhall take the liberty to condemn, as extremely improper and pernicious : becaufe, by ftimulating the nervous membranes and the *dura mater*, they encreafe fpafmodic ftricture, and confequently the prevailing undue *excitement*; but *blifters* applied at a proper diftance from the head, may, without doubt, be ferviceable, by producing a derivation and a counter ftimulus; thus preternatural fpafm is leffened—the fentient principle is diverted to the newly inflamed part, and morbid accumulations of ferum are evacuated. But in thofe fpecies of the diforder named *nymphomania* or *metromania* et *fatyriafis*, the ufe of *blifters* muft be moft ftrictly prohibited; and indeed in every cafe of madnefs where there is a difpofition to *falacity*, which is a very

common

common concomitant fymptom, and ought to be cautioufly and ferioufly attended to. Indeed, in all cafes, bliftering plafters, before they are applied, fhould be either fprinkled with *camphor*, or a fine piece of muflin fhould interpofe them and the fkin, by which means *firanguria*, or what is infinitely more difagreeable, *priapifmus*, will moft generally be prevented. Two fatal inftances of the exceffive ufe of *cantharides* producing *fatyriafis* are recorded by *Cabrolius Obf. Anat.* 17. And others in the *Ephemerides Germanicæ Curiofæ Decad* 1. Plentiful dilution with almond emulfion prepared with a double quantity of gum arab.—Decoct. Althææ, milk and water, or whey, may, with advantage, accompany them, if neceffary. *In melancholia et mania tranquilla*, when dependant on *collapfe* or *undue excitement*, and where, as is frequently the cafe, the biliary ducts are obftructed—the blood in the fplenic vein grows vifcid, and ftagnates—the pancreatic glands perform their office but fparingly, and the blood in the *vena portarum* is rendered thick and fluggifh—

blifters

blifters muft affuredly be of moft eminent
fervice : for, by encreafing the action of the
mufcular fibres, the torpid folids are excited
to more frequent ofcillations, and the force and
celerity of the circulation is confiderably augmented. They alfo reftore the energy of the
fenforium, and the whole nervous fyftem, when
morbidly affected; and of courfe roufe the
mental faculties when weak, languid, and de-
fponding.

I was defired to vifit a refpectable man, who,
the meffenger faid, had a bad fever. I found
him down ftairs—he was very red in the face
—the fkin hot, with an univerfal yellow or bil-
lious fuffufion—the pulfe remarkably full and
flow, and the fecretions at a ftand. As he obferved a profound filence, I foon underftood the
nature of his complaint. I defired that a bed
might be immediately prepared—I led him
gently up ftairs, and he was quietly put into
it. I prefcribed what medicines I judged fit,
and waited till they were given to him, fuf-
pecting that he would not be prevailed upon to
take

take them unlefs I was prefent, and in this I was right. I then ordered his head to be fhaved, and an acrid *blifter* to be applied toti capiti, and gave other neceffary directions; and early the next morning I found him in his perfect fenfes.

This was a ftrong cafe, manifefting the good effects of *blifters* in *Melancholia* or *Mania tranquilla.* It would have been an excellent opportunity for exercifing the *eye,* as I have already defcribed in the art of *management,* had I been apprized of his diforder, and could I have prefented myfelf to him on a fudden; he then, I am convinced, would have taken his medicines without much, if any, entreaty. It was evident, from the yellow tinge on the fkin, that his complaint was occafioned by fome mental depreffion, morbidly affecting the digeftive powers—vitiating the fluids, and particularly the bile—and caufing obftructions in the *pori biliarii.* On enquiry, I learnt that he had, for fome time, followed the *Methodifts*—that his behaviour fince he had embraced the tenets of
that

that sect, became gradually morose—he wan‑
dered from home by himself—would scarcely
give an answer when spoken to, and his repose
by night was greatly interrupted.

I lately attended a very respectable man, in
consultation with a physician of the first emi‑
nence and abilities, in as strong a marked case
of *hypochondriasis* I ever met with. The *chy‑
lopoitic* organs, and indeed the whole contents
of the *epigastrium* appeared to be so much ob‑
structed and diseased, as to be almost insuffici‑
ent for performing the functions of life; but
the application of *blisters* in this unpromising
case, seemed to be productive of the happiest
effects; and with the assistance of other reme‑
dies together with the unremitting assiduity and
benevolence of the physician above alluded to,
the patient recovered.

In order to lessen the determination to the
brain, and to moderate the *preternatural excite‑
ment* of that organ, which takes place in
Mania furibunda, medicines of the *sedative*
class

clafs fhould be tried, either conjointly with or independent of the other evacuants, according as the exigency or the various circumftances of the cafe may feem expedient to the judicious pradtitioner. Their *fedative* power difcovers itfelf by weakening the energy of the *fenforium* —the adtion of the *genus nervofum*, and confequently of the heart and mufcular fibres. They alfo have a power to leffen the motion of the blood when morbidly augmented—allay inordinate and convulfive agitations, and remove fpafmodic tenfion and conftridture. And as maniacs fuftain wa ching for an almoft incredible length of time, it is requifite that they fhould be exhibited in very large and repeated dofes; otherwife our attempts to procure fleep, or calm the ftorm produced by fo great an *excitement*, will be in vain. It is truly aftonifhing to remark, how flight an effedt is produced even by very confiderable quantities of the moft powerful *fedatives*; for dofes which at other times and in other complaints would dangeroufly difturb the fundtions of the animal eco-

M   nomy,

nomy, and particularly thofe of the nervous fyftem, will, during the violence of a fit of madnefs, be fcarcely productive of the fmalleft change. But as fo great an *excitement,* when accompanied with watchfulnefs, powerfully exhaufts the fyftem, every prudent means ought to be ufed, either to remove it at once, or to moderate its excefs and fhorten its continuance. But in *Melancholia et Mania tranquilla,* where the brain is in a *collapfed* or undue *excited* ftate, *fedatives* fhould be given in moderate dofes; becaufe in that cafe, they operate as ftimulants on the fyftem, and have a power to quicken the heart and veffels—encreafe the heat of the body—rarify the fluids, and exhilarate the mind. As they are capable therefore of producing fuch oppofite effects, their adminiftration fhould be regulated by the hand of an expert practitioner.

Camphor is a medicine that has been for a number of years, and is now in general ufe among phyficians, for affuaging or abating maniacal

niacal fury. *Hoffman* has obſerved and recommended its *ſedative* quality more than any
other writer; he gave it in doſes of ℈ij. *Et-
muller* is very laviſh in its praiſes.   Dr. *Kin-
neir*, in the *Philoſophical Tranſactions*, has recommended *camphor* as an effectual cure for
madneſs, given in repeated doſ·s of ʒſs. *Mead's*
annotator, Sir *Clifton Wintringham*, alſo exhibited this medicine with conſiderable advantages:
he ſays, " Hujus medicamenti vires adverſus
morbos maniacos plurimum valuiſſe, experien-
tia fida, comprobatas habui ; eaſque aliquando
ſucceſſu prorſus ſingulari coronatas notavi."   I
gave it in two caſes of *Mania lactea*, and the
patients recovered; but it is to be obſerved,
that *that* ſpecies of the diſorder is almoſt always to be cured, becauſe it certainly does not
depend on any morbid organic affection ; and
I have exhibited it in other ſpecies of inſanity,
with no good effects whatſoever.   And although
it has been extolled by ſuch eminent men, I
muſt frankly acknowledge, that I entertain a
very indifferent opinion of its virtues in this

com-

complaint. Befides, many inftances have been known of fudden and inftantaneous recoveries, independant of any medicine; on which account the effects of *camphor* in the cure of *Mania* will always be doubtful However, as from experiments, and other circumftances, it appears poffeffed of no inconfiderable degree of *fedative* power; it may be capable of inducing fleep, an effect of principal importance in the cure of madnefs; and it is this circumftance only, that juftifies its exhibition in fuch enormous quantities. An imprudent dofe of *camphor* produces vertigo—coldnefs of the extremities—a fmall and languid pulfe—preternatural drowfinefs—uneafinefs about the præcordia —a cold fweat of the head, &c. And although Dr. *Oliver*, in the *London Medical Journal* for the year 1785, part 2. in a dofe of ℈ij wrought a change on the *fenforium commune*, yet the operation was by far too violent, and the effect, as might be expected, of very fhort duration. *Vinegar* is its beft corrector; therefore, when

given

given in fuch large portions, it may be prepared in the following manner:

    ℞ Camph. ʒj.
      Sacchari puriffimi ℥ ſs.
      Aceti calefacti ℔j. Camphora primum cum paulo
      ſpiritu vinoſo rectificato teratur, ut mollefcat,
      deinde cum ſaccharo, donec perfecte mifcean-
      tur ; denique acetum calefactum ſenſim adde,
      et mixturam in operto vaſe frigefactam cola, ut
      fiat acetum camphoratum.

And befides, that the ſtomach will be better
able to retain very confiderable doſes of *acetated
camphor*; the vegetable acid will alſo be a
means of preventing repletion taking place too
faſt in the ſyſtem. The nervine gums, &c.
may be joined with *camphor* on this occaſion ;
and medicines of the ferrugenous or chaly-
beate claſs, may be with propriety added in
Melancholia.

Opium.——*Opium* is the moſt important
and powerful *ſedative* yet known, and medicine without it would be extremely defective.
                                            With

With refpect to its ufe in *mania* there are many difputes. Some affirm that by its *fedative* properties, it would be more likely to *fix* the difo:der than to *remove* it, and it has been fuppofed to have encreafed the paroxyfm of *fury*, and likewife to have induced ideotifm. Thefe are ftrong arguments, undoubtedly, for its exclufion in the treatment of *madnefs*; and I fancy its ufe is, in general, laid afide. I cannot, however, fay much of its virtues in this diforder from my own experience; and although I do not fubfcribe to the above objections, as to its ufe, yet it is impoffible to be too cautious in inculcating any *general* rules for its exhibition, in a bufinefs of fuch importance and concern. The virtues of *opium* confift in caufing fleep, by calming the motion of the fpirits; for watchfulnefs proceeds from the too quick, or irregular motion of the nervous fluid; and fleep is procured by condenfing the nervous ether; accordingly there muft be contained in *opium*, a certain fpirituous and gummy or infpiffating fubftance, that invifcates the fpirits, and impedes, or in a degree arrefts,

arrefts, for a time, the rapidity of their circulation. If thefe good properties can be made
to anfwer, by diminifhing the irritabi.ity—relaxing the tenfion of the fibræ motrices—re-
folving fpafmodic conftriction, and moderating
the motion of the fluids, and thereby procure
fleep, the very beft advantages have fometimes
been gained. But in order to bring about this
important object in *mania furibunda*, large
and repeated dofes muft be adminiftered. It
would be proper to begin with one grain and
to encreafe the dofe gradually, according to its
operation, cautioufly waiting after each, to fee
the effect. If the *fury* fhould be augmented,
its ufe muft be entirely laid afide. And if fleep
fhould be induced, and the vital powers, on
waking, feem to be diminifhed, fo as to threaten
melancholia, the dofe muft be either moderated,
or the medicine prohibited altogether, or, at
leaft, for fome time. *Camphor* may be con-
joined with it, but not the *acetated camphor*,
becaufe acids deftroy the power of *opium*. In
hypochondriacal affections, or *melancholia*, *opium*
fhould be employed with the greateft referve,

as

as in thofe cafes, there are, as I before had occafion to mention, confiderable and frequently very obftinate obftructions and congeftions in the biliary ducts—vena portarum, &c.—but in *mania tranquilla*, attended with pervigilia, when the abdominal vifcera are evidently free of fuch affections, I am clearly and decidedly of opinion, that *opium* may be given in moderate and regulated proportions, in conjunction with the fœtid gums and fteel, with perfect fafety, and oftentimes with advantage.

Mufk.——*Mufk* is one of the moft powerful antifpafmodics we are acquainted with. When taken in large dofes, either in combination with *camphor* or other fœtid nervines, or by itfelf, it proves an excellent mild diaphoretic, cardiac and gentle *fedative* : and, I am convinced, would be a very promifing medicine in *madnefs*, if it could be procured unadulterated. And we muft lament with Dr. *Wall*, that the criteria of the genuinenefs of a medicine of fuch confequence, fhould be fo ill fettled. Perhaps the ftrength of its odour
would

would beſt determine its goodneſs. The high
price it is purchaſed at, is alſo very much
againſt its having a fair trial made of its virtues
in this complaint, in hoſpitals and mad-houſes.
Muſk has the advantage of *camphor* and *opium*,
becauſe it poſſeſſes no deleterious properties;
and when given in an over-doſe, does not produce any diſturbance or inconvenience to the
ſyſtem, but ſlight nauſea or head-ache. When
it is expedient to adminiſter this medicine in a
large quantity, and by itſelf, I ſhould be inclined to prefer the form of pills; becauſe,
when given in that form, the ſtomach would
not only perhaps be better able to retain very
conſiderable doſes, but in that mode of exhibition, the perfume, which is extremely diſagree-
able to ſome perſons, is not, I think, ſo ſtrong
as in any other. The ſubſequent formula may
ſerve for an example.

R Moſch. orient. opt. ʒij.
  Mucilag. g. arab. q. ſ. dividend. in pilul. xxiv
    capiat iij ter quaterve in die.

N   *Hyoſcy-*

Hyofcyamus, or *henbane*, was formerly efteemed to be a medicine of fuch a noxious nature, that neither the plant itfelf, nor any of
its preparations, were employed as internal remedies till the year 1762; when Dr. *Stork*, of
Vienna, publifhed an account of his having
given, with fuccefs, an extract made from the
leaves of this plant, to patients labouring under
difeafes which had been deemed incurable.
He began with giving dofes of one grain twice
in the day, and gradually encreafed the quantity, till he gave ten, twelve, and even twenty
in the fame fpace of time. Dr. *Bergius* advifes this extract to be made from the frefh
juice; and fays, that he has found it to be an
ufeful remedy in *Mania*, given from one to
five grains for a dofe. Dr. *Home* mentions
his having ufed this extract; and concludes
with obferving, that notwithftanding what Dr.
Stork had faid, it did not appear to him to be
antifpafmodic. Dr. *A. Fothergill*, of *Bath*, has
prefcribed it with fuccefs in two cafes of *Infanity*;
an account of which he publifhed in the firft volume of the *Memoirs of the Medical Society of London*,

don, art. 23d. He began with five grains of the extract night and morning, and gradually increased the quantity to thirty grains, and upwards, in the day. It was found, however, that when more than thirty grains were given in that fpace of time, difagreeable fymptoms were occafioned. I do not find that this medicine has been much tried in this country, nor have I heard of any one having made remarkable cures by its ufe; and the almoft univerfal filence on this head, has made me rather fufpect that it has not been much ufed, or that it has failed where it has been tried. I never prefcribed it in any one inftance myfelf; but fince it has been faid to increafe perfpiration, and induce fleep when opium fails, and that inftead of conftipating the bowels, it rather tends to keep them open, I cannot but think that in time and experience, it will prove to be an ufeful antifpafmodic and narcotic, and of fome confideration in the treatment of infanity.

Errhines and *Sternutatories*. It is obfervable, that the infane are very much addicted to fnuff-taking;

taking; and I do not think that propenfity, under proper regulation, is to be objected to. *Errhines* and *fternutatories* are medicated fnuffs, and may have their advantages in this complaint: for they excellently promote the excretion of mucid lymph fecreted in the glandular pituitary membrane, which lines the cavity of the noftrils, and the finufes of the brain.; and are therefore well calculated to abfterge redundant ftagnated lymph from the anterior part of the head. Thefe incentives to fneezing differ only in their degree of ftrength and power of action; the former of which only gently— but the latter more forcibly ftimulates and excites to an excretory motion. In *Mania furibunda, errhines* would be moft proper prepared of the common cephalic herbs; becaufe, by producing a larger exeretion from the mucous follicules of the fchneiderian membrane, they invite an influx of fluids from the neighbouring veffels, particularly from the branches of the external carotids, and thereby, in fome meafure, empty them. But if there be much plethora of the veffels about the head—for fear

of

of producing congeftions, and other mifchief, evacuations of fome kind fhould precede their ufe. In *Melancholia et Mania tranquilla, fter-nutatories* will be of fervice by agitating the body, and roufing the torpor of the nervous fyftem—by encouraging a more brifk circulation, and conveying energy and vigour to the animal functions. The *Pulvis Sternutatorius Officinalis* may anfwer every purpofe on this occafion.

Having thus delivered what I judged neceffary, as far as regards the internal fyftem of medicine, that may, or may not with propriety be purfued in the treatment of infanity—a queftion of very material import in its determination occurs to us, and therefore deferves a few moments confideration. It very frequently happens that maniacal patients refufe their medicines ; nor can they be prevailed on to take them, either by threats or entreaties. It is not uncommon alfo, for fome practitioners on thefe occafions, to force them, and that too, with very confiderable feverity. Now, in what particular

cafes,

cafes, or under what circumftances, is it proper to ufe compulfion? I am well convinced,
from experience, that fuch practice is every
way prejudicial, and ought not, in any cafe
whatever, to be put in execution. It is not
only attended with difappointment to the practitioner, but with great cruelty likewife towards
the patient. In *mania furibunda*, if poffible,
it rather encreafes the *furor*; and in *Mania
tranquilla*, it often times occafions it, becaufe
there is no one circumftance in the treatment
of the infane fo offenfive to them, as *forcing
remedies*: befides, the art and advantage of
government, after this violence, is never to be
acquired; and if you had any authority over
them before, you muft confider it now, as entirely loft: and as on thefe occafions, they
never forget or forgive, their utmoft revenge
may be expected, whenever an opportunity
prefents itfelf. Indeed I hold this practice in
fuch utter abhorrence, that I fhall totally de-
cline explaining the mode of exercifing it.

The

The application of *cold* more generally to the fyftem, is a remedy of principal importance. *Cold* affects us by its *fedative* power in its firft operation: whether its confequent effect arifes from the conftriction which it induces on the veffels, or from its reaction on the *fenforium*, I am unable to determine. There have been inftances of maniacs cured by efcaping from their keepers, and laying feveral hours in the fnow. This complaint, we are informed, has been cured by putting a bonnet of *fnow* on the patient's head, which has brought on fleep, and thus, a change in the fyftem, ending at laft in a perfect cure. Dr. *Cullen* alfo informs us, that benefit has been received in maniacal cafes from the application of *ice*, as well as *fnow*, to the head; and from the ufe of what he calls the noted *clay cap*; but at what period, and in what part of the globe this practice prevailed, I am at a lofs to conceive. The idea is certainly plaufible, and I fhould be of opinion, that it would bid fair to fucceed in *Mania furibunda*, if it were purfued with earneftnefs and affiduity. The ancients were accuftomed

to

to pour *cold water* on the patient's head: the moderns have ufed the *cold bath.* " Capiti, nihil æque prodeft, atque aqua frigida." *Celfus, lib* 1. *cap.* 6. *Mercurius,* the fon of *Helmont,* in his treatife *de Homine,* informs us, that this method of curing mad people was tried in *England* with fuccefs, by a Mr. *Robertfon. Baglivi* obferves, " that mad people have been cured, by being ducked in water after the fame method with thofe bit by a mad dog, whofe only cure confifts in a repeated immerfion." *Bagl. Prac. Phyf.* p. 84. *Van Helmont* mentions an inftance of a man who was going to be bathed in the fea, but efcaped from the carriage, and was cured by plunging himfelf into a pond, where he continued till he was nearly drowned. This circumftance firft induced him to recommend *cold bathing. Boerhaave* advifes this practice to be pufhed fo far as almoft to drown the patient. It may have the fame effect as a *deliquium,* occafioned by bleeding; it may fufpend the intellectual powers for a time; but it is morally impoffible to afcertain the precife time a perfon can remain

under

under water, and be afterwards recovered; on which account, *Boerhaave*'s practice must at once be highly imprudent and dangerous. Attention to the temperament of the patient is more particularly neceffary with refpect to the application of *cold*. This remedy is more peculiarly fuited to the *fanguine* conftitution; but even in the *melancholic*, when the madnefs arifes to a degree of fury, it may be ferviceable—but in degrees inferior to this, it may be very prejudicial, by encreafing the rigidity and drynefs of the fibre, peculiar to that temperament. This rigidity is eafily difcovered by the hardnefs, crifpature, and dark colour of the hair; and in thofe fpecies of *hypochondriac* complaints, attended with heat and unfound vifcera, *cold bathing* would be extremely injurious. If the patient be very much averfe to the operation, I do not fee how it can conveniently, or with advantage, be effected by compulfion; and in this predicament, you run exactly the fame hazard of lofing authority, if you before poffeffed it; as in *forcing medicines*; and befides, what is of principal impor-

O   tance,

tance, the immersion in that operation can never be sudden, and by surprise. I should therefore, were I to practice much in this complaint, prefer the *shower bath*; the patient then may be shocked unawares, and the operation be continued for a greater length of time, even so as to fatigue him, and by that means probably induce sleep. The theory of *cold bathing* may be better understood by consulting *Bellini*, Sir *John Floyer*, Doctors *Bernard*, *Wainwright*, *Burton*, &c.

Warm bathing is more particularly indicated in the *melancholic* temperament, and in those cases attended with a too springy and tense fibre. By the use of the *warm bath*, the rigidity of the solids is mollified—spasmodic constriction is removed, and the vessels are rendered more flexible—dilatable and permeable; and by fatiguing the patient, so as to occasion *syncope*, sleep, in case of pervigilia, might be induced. The *vapor bath* would answer the same end, and I am of opinion, would be more preferable in this disease; because the patient might with

much

much greater convenience be removed from, or continued in the operation, according to the effect it produces. *Cælius Aurelianus, Aretæus Cappadox, Galen,* and *Alexander Trallian,* have all fpoken of it. *Hoffman* alfo infifts ftrongly upon the ufe of this remedy. *Celfus* has not mentioned it, which is fingular. However, it requires much fkill in determining the neceffity of *cold* or *warm bathing* in this difeafe.

The *pedi et manuluvia,* upon the principle of revulfion, may have their good effects, and may with fafety be ufed morning and evening, or oftener, in every fpecies of infanity, and in each temperament of the conftitution, whether fanguine or melancholic. I have more than once or twice known this practice in low nervous fevers accompanied with obftinate watchfulnefs, and an hot dry fkin, bring on fleep— a fine moifture on the furface of the whole body, which proved critical.—" Licet autem pediluvia tantum infimis et extremis corporibus admoveantur, eorum tamen virtus longe lateque fe diffundit et graves in remotis etiam

partibus

partibus morbos levat. Dum enim humore
illo callido foventur pedes, nervofæ, tendinofæ,
ac mufculofæ in iis fibræ ex quibus intercur-
rentibus vafis coagmentati funt, laxantur, remit-
tuntur, pori et tubuli antea conftricti amplian-
tur, et impetus fanguinis ad inferiore derivetur,
&c."—*Hoff.* tom. 3. fect. 11. cap. 10. The
manuluvia well materially affift the other, by
caufing a derivation from the head, and alfo
by inducing fatigue. The partial ftimulus of
heat, like that of cold, produces chillinefs, attended with rigor on firft putting the feet in
hot water, and may be explained, by its con-
tracting, in its firft operation, the fmall cuta-
neous veffels.

External applications to the head (capite prius
derafo) may prove beneficial: fuch as, *aq. rofar.
et acet. vinof. vel aq. Hungaric. et aq. diftillat.
tepid. commixt.—Spir. vin. rect. vel fpir. vin.
camph. vel fpir. lavend.* by themfelves or mixed
in a due proportion *cum aceto*; becaufe fome
parts of them may not only pervade the epider-
mis—cutis—mufcles—pericranium, and the
exterior

exterior perioftium, but alfo pafs to the dura mater, by means of thofe fibres and veffels which that membrane fends through the futures of the fkull to the pericranium. It would be proper to well rub the head with a coarfe cloth, or flefh brufh, previous to the fomentation.

Friction.——" A phyfician ought to be fkilled in many things, efpecially in the nature of *friction.*"—*Hippocrat. de Articulis,* § ix. *Melancholia et Hippochondriafis,* are chronical complaints, and moft commonly attended with two defects, to which the phyfician ought to pay a principal regard, viz —that the folids have loft their proper tone, and that there are obftructions in the vifcera : The intention then muft be to ftrengthen the too much relaxed folids, and remove the obftruction. For this purpofe *Hippocrates* recommends *friction,* and explains its conditions and effects (Εν τῶ χαῖ ἰητρειόν) in thefe words : *Strong friction,* fays he, braces—*gentle friction* loofens—*much friction* diminifhes—and *moderate friction* increafes
the

the flesh. The great master gave no further
explication, as he often wrote in such a manner, as to be understood by those only, who
had made a progress in the art. But *Galen*
has left us a most elegant comment on these
words, wherein he sufficiently explains the sense
of *Hippocrates*. " Soft or gentle *friction*
loosens, or resolves those parts that are braced,
or constipated. Those parts are said to be
braced, or constringed (by *Hippocrates*) that do
not easily move, by reason of some dryness,
cold, inflammation, schirrus, tension, repletion,
or weight. In his second book of preserving
health, where he disputes at large on this matter, against *Theon* and others, no words can
more properly express the nature of obstruc-
tion than these do. *Asclepiades*, as we learn
from *Celsus*, spent the greatest part of a treatise
on the subject of *friction*, of which he claimed
the invention; and, as *Celsus* himself acknow-
ledges, he gave in it more powerful and dif-
tinct precepts, where and how, in what cases,
and in what manner, *friction* was to be applied, than had been done by any of the
ancients.

ancients. *Aretæus* has difplayed great judgment on this fubject, in his beautiful Hiftory
of Chronical Diftempers. This author of fo
great authority, if we may credit the beft cri-
tics, borrowed moft of his fyftem from the
writings of *Hippocrates*, and is, on that account, efteemed his exact and faithful com-
mentator. If it was neceffary, authorities
upon authorities, both ancient and modern,
might be cited, proving the efficacy of *friction*,
as a deobftruent, &c. in all chronical complaints, but more efpecially in *melancholia
et hypochondriafis*, where there are, in general,
fuch obftinate obftructions in the cæliac and
meferiac veffels, &c. *Boerhaave* often lays the
ftrefs of the cure, in moft chronical diforders,
on this remedy. It had been an eafy matter
to have accounted for the effects of *friction*,
from its *phyfiology*; as it accelerates the motion
of the blood in the extreme veffels, and fo proves
a ftimulus, diffolves its vifcid particles, pro-
motes perfpiration, &c. The *hypogaftrium*
fhould be rubbed with warm, dry, coarfe flan-
nel,

nel, every morning and evening, continued for half an hour; two affiftants relieving each other. If there are hard knobs to be felt, or fhould the abdominal fibres and mufcles be very tenfe, *ol. olivar. camphorat.* may be rubbed in with a good intention.

Mufic.——The waves or undulations of the air, occafioned by the ftriking of a mufical in-ftrument, give the fibres of the brain, by the communication of the auditory nerve, thofe percuffions or vibrations, which render founds perceptible at the common *fenfory*, and diftinctly audible and intelligible to the mind, according to the degrees and variety of impreffions made on the *genus nervofum.*

> " Let there be *mufic!* Let the mafter touch
> The fprightly ftring, and foftly-breathing flute;
> Till harmony roufe ev'ry gentle paffion !

ROWE.

The ufe of *mufic* in difeafes, particularly thofe of the mind, is of very antient date; it was the *Nepenthes* of the Gods, to heal the wounded

wounded fpirit. Its power in maniacal complaints, was early and well known; even in
the Jewifh days: as appears from 1ft *Sam.*
chap. 16. where the cure of *Saul,* whofe difeafe was evidently *melancholia,* was effected by
the influence of *David's lyre.*

> " Ceafe your cares: the body's pain
>   A fweet relief may find:
> But gums and lenient balms are vain
>   To heal the wounded mind.
> On every ftring foft breathing raptures dwell,
>   To footh the throbbings of the troubl'd breaft;
> Whofe magic voice can bid the tides of paffion fwell;
>   Or lull the raging ftorm to reft."

Brown's Cure of Saul.

And again:

> " Thus *David's lyre* did *Saul's* wild rage controul,
> And tune the harfh diforders of the foul."

Cowley.

Baglivi fays, " thofe who are forrowful,
angry, or affected with other paffions of the
mind, are excited to chearfulnefs and joy, by

P

the

the gentle and agreeable harmony of *mufic*; and by a continuance of the fame, are lulled afleep." I muft take notice of a paffage of *Alexander ab Alexandro Dier. Genial.* lib. 6. cap. 5. " *Afclepiades* made ufe of nothing more than the *mufical* harmony and concert of voices, in curing frentical perfons, and fuch as were difordered in the mind."

> " *Mufic* the fierceft grief can charm,
> And fate's fevereft rage difarm :
> *Mufic* can foften pain to eafe,
> And make *defpair* and *madnefs* pleafe :
> Our joys below it can improve,
> And antedate the blifs above."
>
> Pope.

The Conqueror of the World was fubdued by the exquifite touches of *Timotheus.*

> " *Timotheus* to his breathing flute,
> And founding lyre,
> Could fwell the foul to rage, or kindle foft defire."
>
> Dryden.

Slow,

Slow, foft, melting ftrains diffufe over the foul an inexpreffible fweetnefs.

" Tange *lyram* digitis animi dolor omnis abibit,
Dulcifonum reficit triftia corda melos."

If thofe who have the direction of *mufic* in maniacal diforders, happen to underftand the *theory* of that fcience, there will be a greater probability of fuccefs, than if it be introduced injudicioufly; for fuppofing the brain to be *collapfed*, or unduly *excited*, or in a ftate of morbid irritability, there muft be fuch an accordance or reciprocation between harmony and the prevalent ftate and affection of the brain, as to occafion a preponderancy in favour of the afflicted. A confiderable fhare of knowledge in *mufic*, then, will be requifite, to felect thofe compofitions and inftruments, and that arrangement of the inftrumental parts, as may, with an exact correfpondence with the *pathos animi*, attract and fafcinate the attention, and influence the temper of the animal fpirits. It will be neceffary likewife to determine whether

the

the *mufic* fhould be performed in the prefence of th e tient, and by furprize; or whether it fhould fteal on the ear, and from a diftance; and whether it fhould be executed in the *alle-gro, andante,* or *dolce—largo* or *prefto* time ; and whether the tone fhould be *forte* or *fortiffimo—* or *piano* or *pianiffimo.* This muft be regulated by the feelings of the patient, which may eafily be afcertained by attentive obfervation to the modulations and ftyle of compofition, which feem to affect him moft fenfibly on the firft performance: and this laft circumftance, will be a rule for judging of the propriety of re-peating or continuing the experiment. And I am ftrongly of opinion, that from this remedy, under the direction of a fkilful phyfician, and provided he is an *amateur* in *mufic,* and the patient has the power of judging of harmony, many important benefits would be derived.

Thus far as to the *therapeutic* branch of the fubject; and if the difeafe will not yield to any of the foregoing remedies, we may venture to pronounce it beyond the reach of art.

There

There is a very curious and juſt obſervation of Dr. *Mead's*, which he illuſtrates with two caſes; and as they are very remarkable, I ſhall recite the whole, and ſubjoin a tranſlation.

" Attamen illud maxime mirandum eſt in hac aegritudine, quod non tantum ea laborantes aliis morbis immunes ſæpe conſervat; ſed et ubi quemquam occupat illis implicitum, ita quaſi totum hominem ſibi aſſumit et vindicat, ut eos non raro depellat ac profliget."—" But a ſurprizing circumſtance in this diſtemper is, that it not only often preſerves the patient from other diſeaſes; but when it ſeizes him actually labouring under them, it lays ſuch ſtrong claim to the whole man, that it ſometimes diſ-poſſeſſes the body of them."——" Duo, quæ hanc rem confirmant, inſignia exempla me vidiſſe memini. Virginem curabam annos natam circiter viginti, mente ſatis alacrem, corpore nimis imbecillam; quæ ex malo habitu diu protracto in hydropem abdominis inciderat, marceſcentibus interim membris. Cum, remediis quibuſcunque fruſtra tentatis, ſpes nulla
ſalutis

salutis affulgeret; supervenit repente, nescio qua de causa, insania cum maximis anxietati-bus et vanissimis animi terroribus; se enim in judicium vocandam esse ob crimen læsæ majes-tatis, et capite plectendam imaginabatur. In-terea corpus vires acquirere, et ventris tumor subsidere cernebatur; ita ut brevi valentiorem medicinam, utrique morbo convenientem, ferre posse videretur. Idcirco vomitu, purgatione per alvum, et medicamentis, tum quæ urinam cient, tum quæ stomachum juvant, ita res age-batur, ut post aliquot menses mens sana sano cum copore rediret."—" I remember to have seen two remarkable instances of the truth of this observation. One was the case of a young lady, about twenty years of age, of a lively and chearful temper, but weakly constitution; who, from a bad habit of body, fell into a dropsy of the abdomen, with great wasting of flesh. Af-ter trying all methods of cure, to no purpose; when she was past all hopes of recovery, she was, on a sudden, seized with madness, (from what cause, I know not) attended with great anxiety and vain terrors of mind: for she ima-gined,

gined, that fhe was to be apprehended, tried, condemned, and executed, for high treafon. In the mean time, fhe gathered ftrength, and the fwelling of her belly fubfided vifibly: fo that in a fhort time, I judged her able to bear more powerful medicines adapted to her two difeafes. Accordingly fhe was put into a courfe of eme- tics, cathartics, diuretics, and ftomachics; which had fo good an effect, that in fome months fhe recovered perfect health of mind and body."

" Alter, quem dixi, morbus, a priore quo- dam modo diverfus, virginem etiam afflixit; quæ annum agens vicefimum et octavum fputo fanguinis, ex pulmone cum tuffi perpetuo fere prorumpentis, vexabatur. Itaque miffus eft e brachio copia fatis larga fanguis, altero quoque die, ad quinque aut fex vices. Minuebatur hinc, non tamen ceffabat malum; et tranfactis duobus menfibus, fupervenit febris hectica, fiti, calore, et nocturnis fudoribus comitata; cum fumma macie, vifcidæque ac tenacis materiæ frequenti exfcreatione, quæ ex faucium et pul- monis glandulis ferebatur, intermixtis hic illic

puris

puris flavi portiunculis. Inftabat jam vera
phthifis, et mors præ foribus adeffe videbatur.
Ægra igitur de animæ falute folicita effe cœpit.
Præfto erant facerdotes, qui cum viam ad cæ-
lum munire deberent, afperam contra et diffici-
lem illam monftrabant, cum precibus, jejuniis,
animique angoribus calcandam; quafi nimi-
rum vitæ futuræ felicitas infelicitatibus et ærum-
nis præfentis vitæ tota effet redimenda. Quid
tandem fit? Mifellam, facris terroribus victam,
brevi invafit religiofa dementia; nocte dieque
oculis obverfabantur dæmonum fpecies, flam-
mæ fulphureæ, et pœnarum apud inferos æter-
narum horrendæ imagines. Ab hoc autem
tempore evanefcere indies cœperunt, quæ morbus antecedens fecum attulerat, incommoda;
decrefcere calor febrilis, fputum fifti, minui
fudores, et habitus totus ita in meliorem verti,
ut, quo minus mens corpori regendo par erat,
eo magis vires officiis vitæ fufficere viderentur.
At paucos poft dies prorfus melancholia evafit.
Morbus igitur exinanitionibus, prout vires ferre
poterant, et idoneis remediis ita oppugnabatur,
ut fanitatis integræ fpes aliqua oftenderetur.

At,

At, proh dolor! poſtquam tres menſes fere
ſunt elapſi, febre heɛ̃tica cum pulmonis exul-
ceratione reverſa, tabe confecɩ̃a periit meliori
fato, ut viſa eſt, digna puella."—" The other,
ſomewhat different from the foregoing, was
alſo the caſe of a beautiful young lady, who
was, in the twenty-eighth year of her age, ſeized
with a violent cough and ſpitting of blood. For
which ſhe was blooded plentifully in the arm,
every other day, five or ſix times. This dimi-
niſhed the violence of the ſymptoms, but did
not entirely remove them: and in two months
a hecɩ̃ic came on, attended with thirſt, heat,
and night ſweats—together with great waſting
of fleſh, and frequent ſpitting of tough ſlime,
from the lungs and throat, interſperſed here
and there with ſmall portions of yellow puru-
lent matter. Now ſhe was running into a
true pulmonary conſumption, and death ſeemed
to be at the door. Whereupon the patient
began to be anxious for the ſalvation of her
ſoul. She was immediately viſited by her ſpiritu-
al guides; who, inſtead of quieting her conſci-
ence, and raiſing her hopes, ſtrongly inculcated,

Q   that

that the way to Heaven was rugged and difficult, and not to be paſſed without faſting,
prayer, and anguiſh of mind: as if the happi-
neſs of the life to come was not to be purchaſed
but by the unhappineſs and miſeries of this life.
But obſerve the event. The miſerable young
lady, overpowered by ſacred terrors, was ſoon
ſcized with religious madneſs. Night and day
ſhe ſaw the appearance of devils, ſulphureous
flames, and other horrid images of everlaſting
tortures of the damned. But from this time, the
ſymptoms of the original diſeaſe began to abate,
the febrile heat decreaſed, the ſpitting ſtopped,
the ſweats grew leſs; and her whole habit was
ſo much changed for the better, that the bodily
ſtrength ſeemed to become more adequate to
performing the funĉtions of life, in proportion
as the mind grew leſs capable of governing
the body. But in a few days ſhe grew quite
melancholic. Wherefore the diſeaſe was treated
by evacuations, proportioned to her ſtrength,
and other proper medicines; which ſeemingly
had ſo good an effeĉt, that there appeared ſome
hopes of a perfeĉt cure. But alas! towards
the

the end of the third month, the hectic and ul-
ceration of the lungs returning, this charming
virgin died consumptive, who seemed worthy
of a better fate.' *Mead de Insania*, cap. 3. p. 74.
——Dr. *Withering* in his account of the fox-
glove, gives two instances, case 24, in 1779, and
34, 1780, of other diseases supervening insanity ;
and with remedies for those, the patients were
releived of both. The late truly celebrated
Dr. *Monro* in his Remarks on Dr. *Battie's*
Treatise of Madness, takes notice of an observation made by the physician of *Bedlam*, who
preceded him, that an intermittent fever coming
upon a madness of long standing, had cured it ;
and of this, Dr. *Monro* says in his publication,
he had seen two or three instances, and one
of them a man who had been extremely mad
for three years. The experienced Dr. *Perfect*
in his Select Cases of Insanity, recites one or
two instances, to demonstrate the interchange-
able relation between insanity and other disorders, and their happy conclusion. *Critical
evacuations* sometimes terminate madness. *Fo-*

Q 2   *restus,*

reſtus, lib. 10. obſ. 24, cured a woman that
grew mad upon ſuppreſſed catamenia, by opening a vein. *Hippocrates Aphor.* 6. 21, ſays,
that if *varices* or the *hæmorrhoids* happen to
mad people, their madneſs is brought to a
criſis. Maniacal complaints have likewiſe been
known to yield to *dyſenteries* and *diarrhœas.*
Puſtles—ulcers, and a ſupervening unſeemly
itch, ſometimes reſembling an *elephantiaſis,* have
done the ſame. An author who tranſlated the
London Practice of Phyſic, contained in the
firſt part of the *Pharmaceutice Rationalis* of
Dr. *Willis,* in the year 1685, and ſubſcribes
himſelf *Eugenius* Φιλατρ☾, ſays, " ſometimes
a *fever* has cured ſome *fools* and *ſtupid* perſons,
and has rendered them more acute." *Huar-
tius* relates, " that a certain *fool* in the court of
Corduba, being affected with a *malignant fever,*
arrived in the height of the diſeaſe to ſo great
an acuteneſs of judgment and diſcretion, that
he put the whole court in admiration, and for
the remainder of his life, continued a very prudent perſon." There is a moſt aſtoniſhing inſtance

ftance in *Bonetus* of a mad patient's being
cured by the *transfusion of the blood of a calf*.
Although the cafe is very long, yet, on account
of its fingularity, I fhall infert the whole of it.
" A patient, thirty-four years old, feven or
eight years ago, became mad, upon a difappointment in Love, where he had conceived
an hope of a vaft fortune. The firft exorbi-
tance was very violent, and lafted for ten
months, without any lucid interval; but afterwards, recovering his right mind by degrees,
he was married. But before he had been
married a year, he relapfed, and has divers
times, for thefe fix or feven laft years, returned
to his right mind. But it is to be obferved,
1. That that indifpofition never lafted lefs than
eight or ten months without any relaxation,
notwithftanding all that could be done. 2.
That a perfon of fame undertook to cure him,
and ufed venæfection in the feet, arms, head,
even till eighteen times, and bathed him forty
times; to fay nothing of applications to the
finciput, and potions: but inftead of amending,
the difeafe feemed to be made worfe by thefe
remedies:

remedies: his phrenſie was always periodical, and never remitted but by little and little; and the remiſſion happened rather when nothing was done to him, than when he was toiled with medicines. Laſt of all, about four months ago, he relapſed into a *delirium* in a place about twelves miles diſtant from *Paris*; where he was ſhut up, yea tied with bands. But, notwithſtanding all the care, he one time got looſe and eſcaped, being quite naked, and ran directly to *Paris*, on a dark night. *D. Montmorius*, being moved with pity, reſolved to get him into one of the hoſpitals, but withall thought of transfuſion, of which ſome experiments had been already made: but as to the cure of ſo great a raving, we did not think our ſelves ſufficiently inſtructed by experience to dare to promiſe it; and our conjectures went no farther than to think that perhaps the freſh *bloud of a calf* might aſſwage the heat and ebullition of his bloud, if it were mixed with it. Therefore, on the ninteenth of *December*, *D. Emereſus* opened the *crural artery of a calf*, and made all the neceſſary preparations; and

having

having let ten ounces of bloud out of a vein in
the right arm of the patient, we could transfufe
into it no more than about five or fix ounces
of the calf's bloud, becaufe his violent pofture,
and the crowd of fpectatours interrupted us.
In the mean while the patient, as he faid, felt
a great heat in his arm and armpits, and per-
ceiving him going to fwoon, we prefently ftopt
the bloud that was a flowing in, and clofed up
the orifice. Yet after two hours he ate his
fupper; and though he was dull and fleepy
betwixt whiles, yet he paft that night over
with the ufual exorbitances: yet the next
morning we found him lefs raving, whence we
believed, that by repeating the transfufion there
would a greater alteration be made in him:
therefore we prepared our felves to repeat the
transfufion at fix a clock in the evening, in the
prefence of many fkilfull phyficians, *Pourdelot,*
Lallier, Dodar, de Bourges and *Vaillant*: But
becaufe the man feemed to be very lean, and
it was not probable that his bloud offended in
quantity, after having fpent three or four days
without fleep or refrefhment, in the cold, running

ning naked about the ſtreets, we onely took two or three ounces of bloud from him at this time; and after we had placed him in a convenient poſture, we performed this ſecond transfuſion in his left arm more plentifully than we had done before: for, conſidering the bloud that remained in the calf after the operation, the patient muſt needs have received more than a pound of bloud. As this ſecond transfuſion was larger, ſo were its effects quicker and more conſiderable. Aſſoon as the bloud entered into his veins, he felt the ſame heat all along his arm and in his armpits which he had done before: his pulſe was forthwith raiſed, and a while after we obſerved a great ſweat ſprinkled all over his face. His pulſe at this moment was very much altered; and he complained of a great pain and illneſs at his ſtomach, and that he ſhould be preſently choaked, unleſs we would let him go. The pipe whereby the bloud was derived into his veins, was preſently drawn out, and while we were buſied in doing up the wound, he vomited up what he had eat before, and beſides, evacuated

cuated both by urine and fæces : by and by
he was laid in his bed, and after he had for two
hours fuftained much violence, vomiting up
divers liquours which had difturbed his ftomach, he fell into a profound fleep about ten
a clock, and flept all that night without inter-
miffion till eight a clock the next day, being
Thurfday. When he awaked he feem'd won-
derfully compos'd and in his right mind, ex-
preffing the pain and univerfal wearinefs that
he felt in all his members. He evacuated a
large glafs full of fuch black urine, that you
would have faid it had been mixt with foot :
he was fleepy all that day, fpake little, and defired that he might be fuffered to be quiet : he
alfo flept well all the next night. Making
water on Friday morning, he filled another
glafs with urine that was altogether as black as
that he made the morning before. He bled a
pretty deal at the nofe, and therefore we
thought it convenient to take from him two or
three porringers of bloud. In the mean time,
his wife, who had fought him from one city to
another, came to *Paris* ; and he, as foon as he

R   faw

faw her, rejoiced greatly, and related to her with great conftancy of mind feveral chances that had befallen him as he wandred about the ftreets, &c. He is now a very quiet fpirit, minds his bufinefs very well, fleeps long without interruption, though, he fays, he has fometimes confufed and troublefome dreams." Here is the conclufion of this moft wonderful cafe. And it proceeds, " This ftory is taken out of an epiftle of *J. Denys*, Doctour of Phyfick and Profeffour of Phylofophy and Mathematicks at *Paris*, concerning transfufion of bloud and infufory chirurgery."

Upon reviewing and contemplating therefore the preceding doctrine and cafes; and at the fame time confidering the generally perverfe and obftinate, as well as the highly deplorable nature of the complaint; and alfo bearing in mind, that the infane are feldom fubject to epidemic, or other diforders, and that madnefs is worfe than death: after an attentive and folemn confideration of thefe particulars, would it be prudent or juftifiable to fuperinduce, by

any

any mode that is moſt practicable, another diſeaſe, on the principle, that the body, by being relieved of the one, might be diſpoſſeſſed of both?

I proceed now to conſider the unhappy ſufferer as conſigned to a dwelling, ſuited to the reſidence of thoſe perſons, who labour under the ſoreſt of all human calamities—a public or private *mad-houſe*. The idea of a *mad-houſe* is apt to excite, in the breaſts of moſt people, the ſtrongeſt emotions of horror and alarm; upon a ſuppoſition, not altogether ill-founded, that when once a patient is doomed to take up his abode in thoſe places, he will not only be expoſed to very great cruelty; but it is a great chance, whether he recovers or not, if he ever more ſees the outſide of the walls. The ſubject of *private mad-houſes* requires ſome conſideration. The conduct of public hoſpitals or inſtitutions, for the reception of lunatics, needs no remark: the excellence in the management of them, is its own encomium. We will con-

R 2   ſider

fider *private mad-houfes* then, as kept and fu-
perintended by two different defcriptions of
perfons. Firft, thofe houfes which are under
the immediate infpection and management of
regular phyficians, or other medical men—or
clergymen. Secondly, thofe houfes which are
under the direction and care of men, who have
juft pecuniary powers fufficient to obtain a li-
cence, and fet themfelves up keepers of *private
mad-houfes*: affuring the public, in an adver-
tifement, that the patients will be treated with
the beft medical fkill and attention, &c when
at the fame time, they are totally devoid of all
phyfical knowledge and experience, and in other
refpects extremely ignorant, and perhaps exceedingly illiterate; and probably without one
qualification for fo important an undertaking.
It will not admit of a moment's hefitation
therefore, to which of thefe two characters we
would entruft an infane friend. In the care
of the firft defcription of men, we may reafon-
ably, and I will venture to fay, fecurely truft,
that the afflicted will be judicioufly and ten-
derly

derly treated; and alfo managed by fervants felected and inftructed with fuch judgement, as will make them as zealous of their own character and reputation, as of the honour of their employer. In fuch hands we may place an implicit confidence; and a perfect affurance, that in fuch an abode, dwells nothing offenfive or obnoxious to humanity—here, no greedy heir, no interefted relations will be permitted to compute a time for the patient's fate to afford them an opportunity to pillage and to plunder. But fuch dwellings are the feats of honour—courtefy—-kindnefs—gentlenefs—mercy; and *whatfoever things are honeft and of good report.* But in thofe receptacles for the unhappy maniacs, as are mentioned in the fecond place, it cannot be fuppofed that any very great advantages in favour of the patient, can be hoped for, or obtained; when compaffion, as well as integrity, in thofe houfes, is oftentimes to be fufpected: this truth is as notorious as it is lamentable. In *September*, 1791, in moft

or

or all of the public newfpapers, appeared the
following article:

" *MAD-HOUSES.*

Notwithftanding the recent regulations,
there are many private mad-houfes in the
neighbourhood of the metropolis, which de-
mand a very ferious enquiry. The mafters
of thefe receptacles of mifery, on the days that
they expect their vifitors, get their fane patients out of the way; or, if that cannot be
done, give them large dofes of ftupifying liquor, or narcotic draughts, that drown their
faculties, and render them incapable of giving
a coherent anfwer. A very ftrict eye fhould
be kept on thefe *gaolers of the mind*; for if
they do not find a patient mad, their oppref-
five tyranny foon makes him fo."——And in
the papers of the following *December*, this
made its appearance.

"*INSANITY.*

Private mad-houfes are become fo general at prefent, and their proftitution of juftice

fo

fo openly carried on, that any man may have his wife, his father, or his brother confined for life, at a certain ſtipulated price ! The wretched victims are concealed from the inſpecting doctors, unleſs it can be contrived, that they ſhall be ſtupified with certain drugs, or made mad with ſtrong liquors, againſt the hour of viſiting ! There ſhould be no ſuch receptacle as a private mad-houſe allowed ; and the relations and friends of the inſane ſhould be allowed to viſit at all times."——And laſt January the ſubject was again brought forward, in the following paragraph :—" Much to the honor of the Surrey Magiſtrates, they have determined to make a very particular enquiry into the management of a number of private mad-houſes. Some of theſe places, which were originally a refuge for the *inſane* only, are now *penſion-houſes* for thoſe whoſe relations wiſh to be the *guardians of their fortunes, overſeers of their eſtates, and receivers of their rents.*"——Theſe are ſufficient and convincing proofs that ſuch villainy exiſts : but it would have been of much more real ſervice and benefit to the

commu-

community, if the authors of thofe affertions had publicly ftepped forth, and dragged to juftice thofe wretches, who *dare* thus trample on the laws of fociety and humanity : and it is fufficient to roufe the hearts of Britons, to excite and expedite an enquiry into thefe enormities, with a fpirit proportioned to the atrocity of them.   An act, paffed in the fourteenth year of the prefent reign, entitled, An Act for Regulating Mad-houfes.   It fets out in the preamble, " *Whereas many great and dangerous abufes frequently arife from the prefent ftate of houfes kept for the reception of lunatics, for want of regulations with refpect to the keeping fuch houfes, the admiffion of patients into them, and the vifitation by proper perfons of the faid houfes and patients : And whereas the law, as it now ftands, is infufficient for preventing or difcovering fuch abufes :* may it therefore pleafe your Majefty, that it may be enacted ; and be it, &c.   The legiflature had an eye to thefe abufes and improprieties, as appears upon the face of the ftatute ; and a redrefs of thofe grievances was, with a proper fpirit of attention and humanity,

manity, the object of that law: but I am confident, from experience, that the ftrict letter of
it is not adhered to, which undoubtedly im-
plies an inadequacy in the ftatute, to the pur-
pofes for which it was enacted: and having
faid thus much; my object at a future feafon
will be, if I am not anticipated in my plan by
talents better fuited to fuch an important undertaking, an alteration and amendment of it.
And I wifh it may be underftood, that I am
not influenced on this occafion by invidious or
malignant motives; for I folemnly avow, that
I entertain no perfonal pique againft any defcription of men whatever: but my aim is,
and always will be, to affert, to the utmoft of
my power, the caufe of thofe poor dementated
creatures; and their caufe, I fhall ever confider,
as the caufe of humanity, and the caufe of
GOD.

I muft add, that *beating* was a practice formerly much in ufe in treating the infane; and
I am forry, and furprized to note, that fome
authors, of very late date, have countenanced

S   fuch

fuch unnatural and brutifh violence. But I will boldly and pofitively venture to declare, that fuch ufage is on no occafion neceffary, felf-defence only excepted : for if maniacs are not to be fubdued by *management*, or by the operation of fear, or both—*beating* will never effect it : but inftead of that, by rendering them more irritable, the fury will be encreafed, and confequently the difeafe lefs likely to be overcome : and therefore, I at once cóndemn this practice, as altogether erroneous, and not to be juftified upon any principles or pretences whatfoever. *Morgagni* mentions the cafe of a patient, who, by order of the phyficians, was bled in the temporal artery : fome little time after the operation, he was found dead. The fact was, the patient having removed the bandages which had been applied to the wounded artery, they were immediately under the neceffity of being replaced, after the lofs of very little blood. However, the perfon to whofe cuftody the maniac had been committed, was fo enraged, that having miferably beaten him, (infano ipfo infaniori)

niori) he threw a very tight bandage about his neck, and departed.—*Morgag. de fedibus et caufis.*

Cafes of maniacal refractorinefs will fome-times occur, which require the ftrongeft and clofeft coertion. On fuch occafions, *chains* and *cords* are frequently employed. A ftrait-waift-coat, which is the beft expedient that ever was invented, will moft generally be fufficient, where the arms and hands only need reftraint. But in very bad cafes, keepers have recourfe to *chains* and *cords*. I once attended an infane patient, the violence of whofe difeafe induced his attendants to tie his legs with cords. When I learnt that he had been for fome days con-fined in this manner, with his legs acrofs, I defired that his bonds might be loofed for my infpection. When, fhocking to relate! the *cords*, by their tightnefs, and the patient's ftrug-gling, had fo lacerated and corroded the tegu-ments, extenfor tendons and ligaments, that a gangrene had abfolutely taken place; and I was not only obliged to have the affiftance of a

furgeon

furgeon of the firft eminence, but alfo to put the patient on an antifeptic courfe of medicine, at a period of the difeafe, I judged extremely unfavourable to fuch a plan : and it was a long time before the fores put on a promifing appearance. It may be proper to remark, that this cafe did not happen in a *mad-houfe*. However, I have it in contemplation, to conftruct an appendage to the ftrait-waiftcoat, which, if it anfwers, will abolifh at once the neceffity of ufing *chains*, and other galling manacles. I mean, when it is compleated, to fubmit it to the private infpection of thofe, who have daily concern with maniacal patients : and if approved on, fhall introduce it to the notice of the public. And I think fome little improvement might be added to the waiftcoat, which will alfo be hereafter taken into confideration.

Before I finally clofe thefe obfervations, I muft offer a few remarks, which could not till now be very aptly introduced.———It is fuppofed

pofed by many, that the *moon* has fome influence in this difeafe: from whence the derivation of the word *lunacy*. But I never obferved
in any maniacal cafe, that the diforder affumed
any particular appearances at any particular
phafes of the *moon*, fo as to make it of confequence in the cure. Dr. *Tyfon*, formerly
phyfician to *Bethlehem* hofpital, remarked, that
the *raving fits* of mad people, which keep the
lunar periods, are generally accompanied with
epileptic fymptoms; and he attefted the fame
to Dr. *Mead*, as a *conftant* obfervation; and he
ufually, on that account, called fuch patients
epileptic mad. The learned Doctor muft undoubtedly have been miftaken. That *epileptic*
fymptoms fometimes accompany madnefs, is
very true: but that they *conftantly* attend thofe
periods, I never could difcover, either by practical obfervation, or ftrict enquiry. Mr. *Wood*,
who formerly kept the Affembly-Houfe at
Kentifh Town, was tried at the Old Bailey for
an highway-robbery, and was acquitted. The
circumftance, however, had fuch an effect upon
him,

him, that he became *epileptic mad*, and died.
I attended him in his indifpofition, with the
late famous and humane Dr. *Monro*. I faw
him repeatedly, and at various times, in his
fits; and I can with confidence aver, that the
lunar periods had no influence whatever, either
in inducing or controuling the *epileptic* fymptoms.

It is impoffible to afcertain the exact period
when lunacy commences; and the diforder,
from whatever caufe it may originate, is always
liable to return, and that in an inftant, or by
gradual fteps, as it may happen. And it may
be further obferved, that a remarkable tendency
to deceit and falfehood accompanies, for the
moft part, this unhappy malady; and this
habit feldom forfakes thofe who have been
afflicted with it, even on a reftoration of reafon,
or what is ufually denominated, a lucid interval. From thefe confiderations, their teftimony
fhould not be admitted in a court of juftice;
nor fhould they be permitted to affix their fig-
nature to any legal inftrument, unlefs the perfons

fons to whofe charge they have been con-
figned, can vouch for the competency of their
intellects.

It is curious, but that very pathos animi,
which may occafion the difeafe, is often to be
difcerned in the vifage of the patient: and in
cafes of religious madnefs, it cannot eafily be
miftaken. I do not affect to be a *Lavater*,
but I do not recollect ever to have been deceived in my *diagnoftic*, in that fpecies of the
complaint.——Madnefs is likewife oftentimes
to be read or *predicted* in the countenance I
have fuccefsfully practifed it; and I am well
convinced, if that branch of the fcience of
phyfiognomy was ferioufly and feduloufly ftudied,
it might be brought to a greater degree of certainty, or even reduced to a fyftem.

It is as worthy of remark as regret, that we can
fcarcely expect *enthufiaftic* madnefs to be releived, much lefs to be cured. And what is
ftill more deplorable, the infane, in that cafe,
are more liable to deftroy themfelves, than in
any other. And not only fo, but they never
                                        lofe

lofe fight of a manner of committing it, when
any particular mode has been determined upon.

> " Come melancholy, for I court thee ftill !
>   As erft come mutt'ring with a downcaft eye,
>   Regardlefs of yon fplendid vernal fky !
> Come ! and of anguifh let me take my fill,
>   Seize my whole bofom, there in fecret kill !
>   Far from the haunts of men with thee I'd fly,
>   Mature my grief, and when refolv'd to die,
>   Fell Suicide, obfequious to thy will,
> Shall hafte with ftagg'ring ftep, and haggard look,
>   Her bowl well drugg'd, her dagger drench'd in blood,
> She all impetuous no delay can brook,
>   But hurries on the deed in defp'rate mood ;
>   To horrid acts woe-haunted minds are driv'n,
>   A wounded fpirit needs the care of Heav'n."

Yet, for our alleviation in fome meafure,
under fuch diftrefs, the all-kind and beneficent
Providence has ordained, that the unhappy object fhould be fubjected to little or no uneafinefs. The obfervation of the *Poet*:

> " There is a pleafure fure in being mad,
>   Which none but madmen know,"

I believe to be juft. This is not only verified
by modern and almoft daily experience, but

is

is likewise confirmed by writers of antient date. I shall first quote a celebrated passage in *Horace*.

———————— Fuit haud ignobilis Argis,
Qui se credebat miros audire tragædos,
In vacuo lætus sessor, plausorque theatro :
Cætera qui vitæ servaret munia recto
More ; bonus sanè vicinus, amabilis hospes,
Comis in uxorem, posset qui ignoscere servis,
Et signo læso non insanire lagenæ :
Posset qui rupem, et puteum vitare patentem.
Hic ubi cognatorum opibus curisque refectus,
Expulit elleboro morbum bilemque meraco,
Et redit ad sese : Pol me occidistis, amici,
Non servâstis, ait ; cui sic extorta, voluptas,
Et demptus per vim mentis gratissimus error.

HORAT. EP. lib. ii. ep. 2.

The case of *Thrasyllus*, as related by *Ælian* in his various *History*, is a further illustration of this doctrine.

Περὶ Θρασύλλȣ παραδόξȣ μανίας.

Θράσυλλος ὁ Αἰξωνεὺς παράδοξον καὶ καινὴν ἐνόσησε μανίαν. Ἀπολιπὼν γὰρ τὸ ἄςυ, καὶ κατελθὼν εἰς την πειραιᾶ, καὶ ἐνταῦθα οἰκῶν, τὰ

T

πλοῖα

πλοῖα τὰ καταίρον]α ἐν αὐτῶ πάντα ἑαυτῦ ἐνόμιζεν
εἶναι, καὶ ἀπεγράφετο αὐτὰ, καὶ αὖ. πάλιν ἐξέπεμπε·
καὶ τοῖς περισωζομένοις καὶ εἰσιῦσιν εἰς τὴν λιμένα
ὑπερέχαιρε. Χρόνες δὲ διετέλεσε πολλὼς συνοικων
τῶ ἀῤῥωςήματι τέτω. Εκ Σικελίας δὲ ἀναχθεὶς ὁ
ἀδελφός αὐτῦ, παρέδωκεν αὐτόν Ἰατρῶ ἰάσαθαι, καὶ
ἐπαύσατο τῆς νόσε ἕτος. Ἐμέμνητο δὲ πολλάκις
τῆς ἐν μανίᾳ διατριβῆς, καὶ ἔλεγε μηδέποτε ἡθῆναι
τοσῦτον, ὅσον τότε ἥδετο ἐπὶ ταῖς μεδὲν αὐτⱳ προ-
σηκέσαις ναυσὶν ἀποσωζομέναις.

Upon very ſtrict enquiry, I never could diſcover, that mad people experience any bodily
pain ; but in general expreſs themſelves perfectly happy and contented. Yet, that they
have ſome ſenſation in the head, I am well
convinced : becauſe I have frequently obſerved
in very ſtrong caſes of *mania furibunda*, that
while the head was ſhaving, or rubbing, they
have been remarkably peaceable, and at the
ſame time ſeemed delighted.

Every man ſhould animate his endeavours
with the view of being uſeful to the world, by
advancing the ſcience which it is his lot to
profeſs

profefs.———With fuch hopes the author undertook, and now difmiffes this work.———And
if a civic crown was formerly beftowed on the
man who faved the life ot a Roman citizen,
furely that perfon may be entitled to equal
commendation, who has *attempted* the refcue
of a fellow creature from a ftate, which is
even more deplorable than death itfelf. And
tho' the phenomena which accompany a pri-
vation of rvafon, and the very flow progrefs
that has been made in the difcovery of remedies, may render opportunities for this exercife
of philanthropy, more defirable than frequent;
yet, let not the fpirit of enquiry be checked,
nor the ardour of humanity be depreffed.———An
infupportable bar may not yet he placed to
further improvement, and very much may be
ftill within the reach of diligent inveftigation.
And as the cure for the greateft part of human
miferies, is not radical, but palliative; we may,
at leaft, endeavour to blunt thofe arrows of
afflicion which we cannot repel, and alleviate
what we cannot remove—remembering always, that the fevereft difpenfations which Providence

vidence vouchfafes to mankind, are for fome wife and good intention; and therefore we fhould never murmur or repine, but wait with patience and refignation, till that period fhall arrive, when the reftitution of all things fhall be completed—all creation regain its original harmony and fplendor, and God fhall be All in All.

F I N I S.